DM ENTRANCE EXAMINATION IN CLINICAL GENETICS

(Includes Important Text, Original solved MCQ's)

Editor :
Dr. M.S. Bhatia (M.D.; MNAMS)
Prof & Head, Department of Psychiatry
University College of Medical Sciences &
Guru Teg Bahadur Hospital,
Dilshad Garden Delhi - 110095.

Contributing Editor :
Dr. (Mrs.) Nirmaljit Kaur (M.D.)
Senior Specialist, Department of Microbiology
Dr. R.M.L. Hospital
New Delhi - 110001

CBS

CBS PUBLISHERS & DISTRIBUTORS

NEW DELHI • BANGALORE (INDIA)

ISBN : 81 39-1367-2

First Edition : 2006

Publishing Director : Vinod K. Jain

Published by :
Satish Kumar Jain for CBS Publishers & Distributors,
4596/1-A, 11 Darya Ganj, New Delhi - 110 002 (India)
E-mail: cbspubs@vsnl.com • Website: www.cbspd.com

Branch Office :
2975, 17th Cross, K.R. Road, Bansankari 2nd Stage, Bangalore-70
Fax : 080-26771680 • E-mail : cbsbng@vsnl.net

Printed at :
Asia Printograph, Delhi

Dedicated to respected teachers
&
beloved students

QUICK MEDICAL EXAMINATION REVIEW

* Comprehensive collection of **Important Text** subjectwise arranged
* Of 3 volumes, **Volume 1** consists of seven subjects of **Basic Sciences** (Anatomy, Biochemistry, Physiology, Pharmacology, Microbiology, Forensic Medicine, & Pathology), **Volume 2** consists of five subjects of **Medical Sciences** (PSM, General Medicine, Dermatology, Psychiatry and Pediatrics) **Volume 3,** consists of seven subjects of **Surgical Sciences** (General Surgery, Orthopaedics, Anaesthesia, , EYE, ENT, Gynaecology & Obstetrics and Radiology)
* Each chapeter has been contributed by an *expert examiner of his field.*
* This book is a cost-effective supplement to the author's comprehensive book on MCQ's i.e. *Quick Medical Examinations Review* (containing over 40,000 MCQ's in 3 volumes)
* **Important Topics** (for MCQ's and undergraduate examinations) in *each subject* has been listed in the beginning. Each chapter contains important factual data, numerous named/signs/syndromes and important points to be remembered.
* There is *no need to underline* a standard textbook for MCQ's as important points to be remembered have been added at the end of each chapter.
* The book contains text from many standard textbooks of each subject.
* This book is presented with the hope and wish to invite fruitful interaction, comments, suggestions and contributions from its readers. This book is a must before any PG Entrance Exam.
* A favourite book for Paper Setters and examinees. This book covers 60% to 99% of MCQ's asked in various examinations
* Edited by: **Dr. M.S. Bhatia (MD; Dip. W.P.A.)** - an experienced teacher and examiner who has worked in three leading Medical Colleges of Delhi (Maulana Azad Medical College, Lady Hardinge Medical College & University College of Medical Sciences) under Delhi University.

A Book by the readers, of the readers, for the readers.

PREFACE

Genetics is a rapidly advancing field. Its new allied branches are coming up. In a competitive examination, more and more emphasis is being laid on these allied disciplines. But most of the standard textbooks of genetics have failed to devote adequate space to these new disciplines.

This book has been written with the aim to outline the major areas of Clinical genetics i.e Factual data, Commonest cause, Basic concepts and *Recent advances.* This book is not merely an addition to the existing list of books on MCQ's but a sincere ambition and an honest attempt to make it a useful and practical companion to both medical graduates and postgraduates. The present book consists of original solved MCQ's from the *Question Banks* of various important examinations (AIIMS, Delhi, PGI etc.), Important text, original solved MCQ's and their explanations. This book is also useful for DM Entrance in Clinical Genetics (in SGPGI, AIIMS etc) and also other entrance examinations. We hope that this will help the candidates in performing better in the examination.

All suggestions for the modification of this book are welcome and will be duly acknowledged.

—Editors

CONTENTS

Preface

Dedication

IMPORTANT TEXT	1—64
ORIGINAL SOLVED MCQ'S	65—110

IMPORTANT TEXT OF CLINICAL GENETICS

IMPORTANT POINTS TO REMEMBER

* DNA absorbs ultraviolet light maximally at the wavelength of **260 nm.**
* Length of DNA in a single human cell is **1.74 metres.**
* RNA chain growth proceeds in **5 to 3 direction.**
* There are **64** possible codons
* Adenine and guanine are purine bases while cytosine, thymine and uracil are pyrimidine bases
* RNA contains AGCU while DNA contains AGCT respectvely..
* **Chargaff rule** states that A/T = G/C.
* The initial codon to be transmitted in m—RNA in eukaryotes is **G-U-A (val).**
* 2 DNA strands are held together by hydrogen bonds.
* DNA has got an important role in directing the synthesis of m-RNA referred to as **transcription**.
* Coffee contains — Caffeine (1,3,7 trimethylxanthine).
* DNA helix is — **Right handed** and held by Hydrogen bonds.
* Z-DNA is —**Left** handed **double** helix.
* Enzyme required to produce double stranded DNA from RNA genome — RNA dependent DNA polymerase or Reverse transcriptase.
* All RNA molecules contain — ACC at 3 terminus.
* **Pseudogenes** are — Genes containing nonsense codons, thus do nt express.
* **Okazaki** pieces — Fragments of DNA attached to an RNA primer with approximately 10 nucleotides.
* **Polymerase alpha** is responsible for — Chromosome replication in nucleus.
* **Polymerase beta** plays role in —DNA repair.
* **Polymerase gamma** replicates — Mitochondrial DNA.
* The energy required for formation of one peptide bond is equivalent to — Hydrolysis of 2 ATP to ADP and 2 GTP to GDP.
* Initiating codon is — AUG (codes for methionine).
* **Puromycin is** — An antibiotic inhibiting protein elongation.
* Mutation involving change of one pyrimidine for another is known as — **Transition.**

* Change of pyrimidine for purine or vice versa is known as —**Transversion.**
* Part of m-RNA removed during protein synthesis is — **Intron.**
* t-RNA contains the anticodon for — **Transcription.**
* DNA polymerase III is the primary DNA-polymerase involved in DNA replication.
* Helicase activity provides single strand templates for replication.
* Eukaryotic replication proceeds bidirectionally from many origins.
* **Replicons** are the basic units of replication. It takes about eight hours to replicate the human genome.
* **'S' phase** in a cell cycle is the phase in which DNA is synthesized.
* Eukaryotes replicate their DNA only once per cell division cycle.
* Most prokaryotic mRNAs are **polycistronic.**
* Most eukaryotic in RNAs are **Monocistronic.**
* RNA polymerases have no other associated enzyme activities.
* Promotor sequences are responsible for directing RNA polymerase to initiate transcription at a particular point.
* **Splicing** is a process by which noncoding sequences are removed to form functional m RNA.
* Codons are group of three adjacent bases that specify the aminoacids of protein.
* Most amino acids are coded by more than one codon.
* Genetic codes are universal.
* **Ricin** is a protein produced by castor beans which inhibitis protein synthesis in eukaryotes.
* **Most common** type of mutation is Base substitution.
* Carcinogenic potential of a carcinogen is estimated by **Ames test.**
* Preferred vector for establishment of genomic libraries is Bacteriophage lambda.
* **Southern blot analysis** is used for :-
  (i) Identifying the number of genes in the genome
  (ii) Forming the basis of Restriction Fragment Length Polymorphism (RELP)
  (iii) DNA fingerprint analysis.
* **Northern blot analysis** is used to detect RNA.
* DNA sequencing can be done enzymatically by **Sanger procedure** and chemically by **Maxam Gilbert procedure.**
* **Unwinding** of DNA is done by Topoisomerase I.
* **'Leucine zipper' motif** is a mediator for binding of regulatory proteins of DNA.

* Proof reading of m-RNA is done by Aminoacyl transferase.
* UV rays causes dimensation of pyramidine.
* The following base sequence and its complementary sequence are palindromic AATT.
* Gene that is involved in transcription but excluded before translation is intron.
* In Gene cloning, **largest** segment is cosmid.
* **Okazaki segment** is used for DNA synthesis.
* Triplex helix is seen in collegen.
* **Okazaki fragments** are short pieces of DNA replicated continuously in the 5'-3' direction.
* **Degeneracy** of the genetic code denotes the existance of multiple codons for a single amino acid.
* **Chargaffs observation** on nitrogen base contents of DNA of all species is that there are equal numbers of 2 and 3 are correct.
* **Post-translational hydroxylation** of uracil forms thymine in transfer RNA.
* In post-transcriptional processing of m-RNA, **"splicing"** refers to joining exons after the removal of introns
* The **melting temperature** (Tm) of DNA is related to the base composition of DNA.
* DNA fingerprint is valuable in investigation of crime and determination of paternity.
* Processing of RNA is the function of **"small nuclear ribonucleoprotein particles** (SnRNP).
* Function of endonuclease cut DNA at specific DNA sequences.
* **Anticodon** is present in t-RNA.
* Histones are activated in gene expression by formylation.
* Analysis of DNA genome is done by **Southern blot test**.
* Anderson's disease is type IV glycogen storage disease.
* **"Jumping genes"** are also called Trypnosons.
* **Leucine zipper motif** is an alpha helical structure in which leucine is regularly repeated.
* In helix turn helix motif, alpha2 and Alpha3 helices are held at 90° to each other by a turn of 4 amino acids.
* A series of loops of chromonemata of polytene chromosome similar in nature to chromosome puffs and in appearance to lampbrush chromosome is **Balbiani's ring.**
* **Ambisence RNA** is a type of mRNA.
* **Chromosome walking** is defining relation of different genes on a long stretch of DNA.

* Alpha and Beta sheet orientations or polypeptide chains were deduced by **Pauling and Corey.**
* The amino acids coded by 6 codons are arginine, leucine and serine.
* **Wobble** is present in tRNA.
* **Chromosomal walking** : In it, a fragment representing one end of a long piece of DNA is used to isolate another that overlaps but extends the first.
* **Pseudogene :** An inactive segment of DNA arising by mutation of a parental active gene.
* During DNA melting, as the bases are separated, absorbance at 260 nm increases.
* The rapidity of growth is proportional to the intensity of the metabolic process is Rubner's law.
* DNA relaxed molecule is when there is **Simple circular** structure.
* Rapid cooling of the denatured DNA fixes it in a permanently denatured state and is called **quenching.**
* Locus for Duchenne muscular dystrophy is **Xp21.2**
* **22q** Chromosome region may be affected in CLL, ALL and meningioma..
* Most normal persons have two M genes, but the **Z gene** is responsible for low production of alpha-1-antitrypsin, a condition associated with familial emphysema.
* Congenital malformation of fetus is DM diagnosed by HbA1AC.

MOLECULAR GENETICS AT A GLANCE

— The **human genome** consists of 3 billion base pairs of DNA with two copies of the double stranded helix in each cell nucleus and mitochondria distributed in 23 chromosomes encoding about 50,000 genes (10% of total DNA).

Note : Genes expressed on mitochondrion are only of maternal origin

— A **gene** is functional unit of DNA from which RNA is copied (transcribed) and, in the case of most human genetic diseases, translated (mRNA) by cellular machinary into a family of proteins in the cytoplasm.

— **Mutations** are variations of DNA that affect the functioning of genes and thereby, the patient, polymorphisms are variations in DNA that do not affect the health or functioning of the organism.

Note : Mutations in germ, not somatic cells, are heritable.

— Advances are greatly influenced by the technology o sequencing (base pairs) : cloning (amplifying a sequenc or fragment of DNA to yield large amounts of the DNA segment).

by —inserting and deleting sequences

—the use of single stranded DNA or RNA sequences (probe) to find comple mentary fragments by hybridization.

—enzymatic amplification of a DNA segment by polymerase chain reaction and the like.

Thus, a disease can be diagnosed by examination of an individual's DNA once the disease is suspected to be present in the patient or a carrier.

Human gene linkage maps are developed by locating genes or nongene DNA sequences to precise site on a chromosome and determining the position relative to each other of individual genes or DNA sequencs on the chromosome.

— **A disease gene can be found by :**

1. The "forward" or "classic" method by identifying a specific defective protein, determining its sequences of amino acids and comparing it to a normal sequence to identify the abnormality, and then isolation, cloning and sequencing in m RNA for the abnormal protein, from which the complementary DNA sequence containing the mutation can be identified.
2. The "reverse" genetic approach, in which in mutated gene is first identified isolated, and sequenced by DNA analysis and subsequently the abnormal gene product (protein) or its absence is determined and its pathophysiology elucidated.

   Genetic disease can be diagnosed by examining DNA from almost any cell of a patient at any time in the life of an individual.

— Many thereapeutic molecular genetic interventions are being developed.

Genetic abnormalities :

Single mutan genes exhibit one of the following pattern of inheritance given below :

Autosomal dominant :

— Here a child of an affected parent has a 50% chance of inheriting the genetic disorder.

Autosomal recessive :

— A child of two heterozygous parents has a 25% chance of inheriting the geneting disorder.

X-linked recessive :

— Each daughter of a carrier has a 50% chance of being a carrier and each son a 50% chance of inheriting the disorder.

X-linked dominant :

— Males and females may be affected but all daughters and no sons of a affected father will be affected.

Multifactorial inheritance :

— It refers to a process in which an abnormality is the result of the additive effects of one or more genes and environmental factors.

Chromosomes and their abnormalities :

— About 1 in 150 newborns have an abnormality in the number or structure of the normally 46 chromosomes in a karyotype.

21 trisomy (Down syndrome, mongolism) is the most frequent autosomal syndrome.

Ther eis high correlation between increasing maternal age and nondisjunction resulting in an extra chromosome.

Translocations (transfer of a segment from one chromosome to another) are the most common structural aberrations. usually the loss or gain of chromatic material is unbalanced or not reciprocal resulting in an abnormal phenotype. **Chromosomes 9,11,13,14,15,21 and 22** are frequently involved.

— Deletions are most commonly associated with **chromosome 4,5, 9** and 11. They result in characteristic C/F that often include **mental retardation.**

— **Breakage of chromosomes** is associated with **neoplastic diseases,** such as leukaemias, and with autosomal recessive disease, such as **Bloom syndrome.**

— About half of chromosome abnormalities involve sex chromosomes : eg
Turner syndrome (45 XO)
Klinefelter syndrome (47 XXY)
Fragile X syndrome

Congenital malformation

About 2% of newborn have major malformations, about half of which are genetic. There are correlations with genetic diseases, chromosomal abnormalities in utero infections, and teratogens, but the causes of > 40% remain unknown.

— Dysmorphology may result deformation or disruption of a developing previously normal structure, in addition to malformation (a primary structural defect arising from a localized error in morphogenesis).

GENETICS

* Transferring DNA fragments to a Nitrocellulose filter is called- Southern blot technique.
* A labelled single stranded DNA used in southern blot technique is called - probe
* Substance usually employed - for labelling the DNA - Phosphorous (P32)*
* Random inactivation of x chromosome is known as - lyonisation
* The incidence of down's syndrome is 1 to 700 live births. (The commonest genetic cause of mental retardation)

* Conditions associated with Down syndrome - Heart disease, leukemia, ALL, endocardial cushion defects, Hirschsprung's disease, annular pancreas.
* The children with down's syndrome are predisposed to
* Simian palmar crease is a feature of - Down's syndrome
* The commonest abnormality in Down's syndrome - Trisomy 21
* The commonest translocation in Down's syndrome 13, 14, 15/21
* Polydactyly is a feature of - Patau's syndrome
* Epilepsy is a feature of - Wolffe's syndrome
* "Rocker bottom feet" are a feature of - Edward's syndrome*, Patau's syndrome.
* Microcephaly is a feature of patau's and cri-du-chat syndromes
* Hypertelorism is a feature of cri-du-chat syndrome. (*It can also occur due to fracture of nasal bones*).
* Hypospadias is a feature of wolffe's syndrome
* The first sex chromosome Aneuploidy described in males - Klinefelter's syndrome*
* The first allosome aneuploidy described in females - Turner's syndrome*
* Coarctation of Aorta is associated with -Turner's syndrome.
* Coarctation of Aorta is more common in males.
* Patent ductus Arteriosus is more common in females.
* The probability of a genetically predisposed person to express the disease is called- Penetrance
* Nephrogenic diabetes insipidus is inherited as - x linked recessive
* The disorder with the maximum heritability is - Schizophrenia (83%)
* The heritability of essential hypertension is 62%
* The heritabilility of coronary Artery disease is 65%
* Gargoylism is a feature of - Hunter's and Hurler's syndromes
* Corneal clouding is a feature of - Hurler's syndrome
* Transabdominal Amniocentesis is ideally done at 16th week of gestation.*
* The main application of cytogenetic Amniotic fluid studies - Diagnosis of Down's syndrome.
* Transcervical chorionic villus biopsy is done at 8 to 10 weeks gestation.
* Southern blot technique - for DNA

  Northern blot technique - for RNA.

  Western blot Technique - for HIV
* **Down's Syndrome :** (21-trisomy; Mongolism)
  * Incidence : 1 in 600-800 live births
  * Presence of extra No 21 chromosome.
  * ↑ Maternal age & nondisjunction

* Characterised by small & round skull, flat facies small nose, short neck, dysplastic ears, oblique palpebral fissures, furrowed tongue (scrotal tongue, clinodactyly, simian crease, Hypotonic muscles with normal jerks).
* Mental retardation
* Eye changes include Epicanthus, hyperelonism, Brushfield spot on iris, cataract, squint, high myopia, nystagmus & keratoconus.
* Associated with duodenal atresia and cardiac spetal defects & ↑ incidence of acute leukemia.

SINGLE MUTANT GENES DISORDERS & PATTERN OF INHERITANCE

PARENTS	CHILDREN		
	Affected	**Carriers**	**Normal**
Autosomal Recessive Inheritance :			
* Autosomal Recessive + Normal	—	50%	50%
* Both Autosomal Recessive	25%	50%	25%
Autosomal Dominant Inheritance :			
* Autosomal Dominant + Normal	50%	—	50%
X-Linked Recessive Inheritance :			
* Normal male + Carrier female	50% sons & 50% daughters	50% daughters	50% sons
* Affected male + Normal female	—	All daughters	All sons
X-Linked Dominant Inheritance :			
* Normal male + Affected female	50% sons & 50% daughters	—	50% sons & 50% daughters
* Affected male + Normal female	All daughters	—	All sons

Edward Syndrome : (18-trisomy syndrome)

* Incidence is 1 in 8000 births.
* Results from trisomy of No. 18 chromosome due to nondisjunction.
* Typical facies with low set ears, micrognathia, high arched palate, webbed neck.
* Muscle hypertonicity, flexion of fingers 92nd overlapping 3rd; Rocker bottom feet, shield chest, joint abnormalities).
* All have cardiac malformation, hypertrichosis, Meckel's diverticulum, cryptorchidism.
* Eyes show unilateral ptosis, epicanthus, corneal & lens opacities.
* Infants die most frequently within the first 3 months of life.
* **Patau's syndrome :** (13 trisomy syndrome)

* Incidence is 1 in 20,000 livebirths.
* Chromosome No. 13 found in triplicate.
* Microcephaly, arrhinencephaly, sloping forehead wide sagittal sutures 7 Fontanelles.
* Eye shows micropht almia, horizontal palpebral fissures, cataract, iris coloboma & retinal dysplasia.
* Harelip with cleft palate.
* Single palmar transverse crease
* Polydactyly with narrow hyperconvex nails.
* Kidney polycystic, hydronephrosis.....renal or ureteral duplication.
* Genital anomalies are cryptochis, bicornuate uterus & double vagina.
* Cardiac defects are PDA, ASD, VSD dextroposition of heart.
* Most infants die in the 1st year of life.

* **Klinefelter's Syndrome :**
  * 47XXY.
  * Incidence is 1 per 1000 liveborn males.
  * Associated with advanced maternal age.
  * Results from a sex chromosome complement that includes 2 or more X-chromosomes & one or more Y-chromosomes.
  * ↑ height; ↑ length of legs, weak growth of facial hair.
  * Female distribution of fat & sexual hair, gynaecomastia, testicular hypoplasia, sterility, subnormal libido.
  * ↑ plasma testosterone levels
  * Mild mental retardation & behaviour disturbances.

* **Turner's Syndrome :**
  * Incidence 1 in 10,000 live female births.
  * 45, X, buccal & other cells are sex chromatin negative.
  * Results from complete or partial monosomy of the short arm of X-chromosomy.
  * Skeletal anomalies include short stature, shieldshaped chest, Cubitus valgus & webbed neck.
  * Infantile sexual development with streak gonads, amenorrhoea, enlarged clitoris & hirsutism & ovary without primordial follicles.
  * Coarctation of aorta & hypertension.

* **COMMONEST**
  * More common features of children with chromosomal abnormalities are -odd facies, abnormal ears, heart & kidney malformations, abnormal hands & feet, simian creases, single crease on 5th finger & low birthweight.
  * The most common type of aneuploidy is trisomy.

* Tests for sex chromatin most often utilize cells scraped from buccal mucosa (buccal smear).
* Somatic abnormalities are more common in the Klinefelter's syndrome when it is caused by chromosomal abnormalities other than 47, XXY.
* The commonest trisomy is Down's sydnrome
* The second common trisomy is Edward's syndrome.
* The commonest autosomal recessive disorder in the West in cystic fibrosis.
* Both males & females are affected in X-linked dominant inheritance but males are often more severely affected.
* The most important clinical indications fo chromosomal study are Congenital malformations (if more than one system is involved) & mental retardation of unknown origin.
* A deletion of the long arm of chromosome 13 (including band 13q 14) is associated with retinoblastoma.
* Clinical signs of chromosome 21 deletions are variatins of Down's syndrome known as 'Antimonogloism".
* is ordinarily the most brightly fluorescent chromosome.
* Most genetic counselling sessins begin with pedigree analysis.
* Husband-wife consanguinity leads to↑ risk of having child with a birth defect (especially autosomal recessive disorder or multifactorial disorder.
* ↑ *risk of autosomal recessive disorders :*
* Tay-Sachs disease..... Ashkenazi, Jewish & French canadian populations.
* β-thalassemia ......Greek, Italian 7 Mediterranean descent.
* Sickle cell disease ..... American & African blacks
* Cystic fibrosis....... Northern European descent.

* In Klinefelter's syndrome a direct correlation is apparent between the ↑ likelihood & severity of mental retardation & ↑ number of X-chromosomes.
* In autosomal recessive inheritane the affected individuals are almost always born in only 1 generation of family.
* In X-linked nrecessive inheritance only males are clinically affected (affected males do not have affected sons but may have affected grandsons born to carrier females).
* 90% of karyotypically abnormal conceptins do not survive pregnancy.
* The long arm of the X-chromosome is associated with mental retardation.
* The older the mother, the greater the likelihood of nondisjunction & trisomy. (Monosomy may result from chromosome loss or anaphase lag).

* Mental retardation is not a feature of Turner's syndrome (but a recent review noted its presence in 18% patients).
* Turner's syndrome shows high ridge count where as Klinefelter's shows low ridge count (dermal pattern of digits)
* The aetiology of about 40% of congenital malformations are unknown.

* **UNIFACTORIAL INHERITANCE**

Autosomal dominant inheritanc

* Dominant trait manifests in heterozygote.
* Every affected person has an effected parent.
* Every affected person who marries a normal person has 1 in 2 chance of having each offspring affected.
* Every normal child of an affected person will have normal offspring
* Males and females are affected in euqal proportions.
* Because of smaller size of moder families, by chance all children of affected individual may be normal by affected

Autosomal recessive inheritance

* Autosomal recessive traits are manifests only in the homozygous state.
* Affected persons have parents who are normal in all outward appearnces.
* In affcted families, each child has 1 in 4 chanc of having a genetic defect.
* When an affected person and a normal person marry their offspring will be normal (in most cases).
* When 2 affected persons marry, all their children will be affected.
* One-quarter (25%) will be affected.
* Consanguinity in the family tree.

X-linked dominant inheritance

* Females are affected about twic as often as males.
* Affected females transmits the disorder to half of her sons and half of her daughters.
* Affected male transmits the disorder to all his daughters and to none of his sons.
* It is more variable and less severe in heterozygous affected females than in hemizygous affected males.

X-linked recessive inheritance

* Predominantly affect males and are transmitted by healthy female carriers. (The defect is carried by women and exhibited by men)
* All female offspring of affected males are carriers. (Affected men can pass the disease only through their daughters).
* In males, amutant gene present on the single X chromosome is always manifest.

* X-linked trait is never transmitted from father to son.
* Male offspring of carrier women have a 50% chance of being affected
* Unaffected males do nto transmit the trait to any offspring.
* Affected homozygous females occur only when an affected male fathers the child of a carrier female.

Hereditary Structural and Functional Traits

Dominant	Recessive
* Curly hair	* Straight hair
* Dark brown hari	* All other colours
* Coarse body hair	* Fine body hair
* Pattern baldness (dominant in males)	* Baldness (recessive in females)
* Normal skin pigmentation	* Albinism
* Brown eyes	* Blue or grey eyes
* Near or farsightedness	* Normal vision
* Brown eyes	* Blue or grey eyes
* Near or farsightedness	* Normal vision
* Normal hearing	* Deafness
* Normal colour vision	* Colour blindness
* Broad lips	* Thin lips
* Large eyes	* Small eyes
* Polydactylism (extra digits)	* Normal digits
* BRachydactylism (short digits)	* Normal digits
* Syndactylism *webbed digits)	* Normal digits
* Hypertension	* Normal blood pressure
* Diabetes insipdus	* Normal excretion
* Huntington's chorea	* Normal nervous system
* Normal mentality	* Schizophrenia
* Migraine headaches	* Normal
* Normal resistance to disease	* Susceptibility to disease
* Enlarged spleen	* Normal spleen
* Enalrged colon	* Normal colon
* A or B blood factor	* O blood factor
* Rh blood factor	* No Rh blood factor

Recognizable Genetic conditions

Unifactorial Disorders

* **Autosomal Dominant**
    * Achondroplasia
    * Facioscapulohumeral muscular dystrophy
    * Familial hypercholesterolemia
    * Gilbert's sydrome
    * Hereditary hemorrhagic telangiectasia
    * Hereditary spherocytosis
    * Huntington's chorea
    * Hyperlipoproteinaemia Type II
    * Idiopathic hypertrophis subaortic stenosis (IHSS)
    * Marfan's syndrome
    * Myotonic dystrophy
    * Neurofibromatosis
    * Noonan's syndrome
    * Osteogenesis imperfecta
    * Polycystic disease of kidneys (adult form)
    * Polyposis colon
    * Porphyria, acute intermittent
    * Retinoblastoma
    * Tuberous sclerosis
    * von Willebrand's disease
    * Autosomal Recessive
    * Albinism
    * Ataxia telangiectasia
    * Crigler-Najjar syndrome
    * Cystic fibrosis
    * Deafness
    * Dubin-Johnson syndrome
    * Familial Mediteraranean fever
    * Fanconi's syndrome
    * Friedrich's ataxia
    * Galactosaemia
    * Gaucher's disease
    * Glycogen storage diseases
    * Hemochromatosis
    * Hereditary emphysema

  (alpha-antitrypsin deficiency)
  * Homocystinuria
  * Hurler's syndrome
  * Limb girdle muscular dystrophy (Erb)
  * Niemann-Pick disease
  * Phenylketonuria
  * Pendred's syndrome
  * Sickle cell anaemia
  * Thalassemia (beta)
  * Tay-Sachs disease
  * Wilson's disease
* **X-linked Dominant**
  * Amelogenesis imperfecta
  * Bipolar depressive psychosis
  * Goltz's syndrome
  * Hypophosphatemia
  * Oral-facial-digital syndrome I
  * Vitamin D resistant rickets
* **X-linked Recessive**
  * Colour blindness
  * Christmas disease
  * Duchenne muscular dystrophy
  * Fabry's disease
  * G6Pd deficiency * Fabry's disease
  * Haemophilia
  * Hunter's syndrome
  * Lesch-Nyhan syndrome
  * Nephrogenic diabetes insipidus
* **Y-linked disorders**
  * Not existing
* ***Multifactorial disorders***
  * Asthma
  * Diabetes mellitus
  * Cleft lip + cleft palate
  * Pyloric stenosis (Congenital)
  * Ankylosing spondylitis
  * Club foot (Congenital)
  * Coronary artery disease

* Hypertension (essential)
* Dislocation of hip (congenital)
* Anencephaly and spinabifida
* Anencephaly and spinabifida
* Peptic ulcer
* Congenital heart disease (all types)
* Epilepsy
* Manic-deprssive psychosis
* Psoriasis
* Thyroid disease

Chromosomal aberrations

Numerical :

* Down's syndrome (94%)
* Kilnefelter's syndrome (85%)
* Turner's syndrome (90%)

Structural :

* Down's syndrome (3%)
* Cri-du chat syndrome
* Wolf-Hirschhorn syndrome

Mosaicism :

* Down's syndrome (3%)
* Klinefelter's syndrome (15%)
* Turner's syndrome (10%)

Chromosomal abnormalities

Monosomy Imbalance Karyotypes — Recognised Clinical Syndrome

Monosomy :

* 45 , x ....Turner's syndrome

(Segmental deficiency)

* 46, xy, 4p - ... Wolf's syndrome
* 46, xy, 5p ... Cri-due-chat syndrome
* 46, X5, 15 q ... Prader-Willi syndrome
* 46, xy, 17 p ... Miller-Dieker syndrome
* 46, xy 18- ... De Gronchy's syndrome
* 46, xy, 18q- ... De Gronchy's syndrome
* 46 xy, 21 q ... Anti mongolism (Gdeletio syndrome I)

Trisomy

* 47, xxx ... (Super female syndromes)
* 476, xxy ... Klinefelter's syndrome
* 47, xxy ... (xxy syndromes)
* 47, xy, +131 ... Patau's syndrome
* 47, xy, +18 ... Edward's syndrome
* 47, xy, +21 ... Mongolism (Down's syndrome)

Partial trisomy :

(Segmental duplication)

* 46, x, t (x; y) ... xx male

Chimerism :

(entire complement chromosomes effected)

* 46, xy/46, xx ... Pseudo-or true hermaphroditism; (Dimor phism of blood cell surface antigens)

Triploidy :

(entire complement)

* 69, xxy ... Hyddrocephaly, Intellectual deficit, syndactyly, cardiac malformation, abnormality of ext. genitalia, and early death

* **Sex Chromosomal Syndromes**

	Syndromes	*Chromosomal No.*	*Sex chromatin*
*	Turner's	45 XO	-
*	Super female	47 XXX	+2BB*
*	Tetra X	48 XXXX	+3BB*
*	Penta X	49 XXXXX	+4BB
*	Klinefelter	47 XXX	+1BB
*	Klinefelter	48 XXYY	+1BB
*	XYY	47 XYY	-
*	True hermaphrodite	46 XX	+
		XY	
	XXXY		
*	Male pseudo-hemaphrodite	46 XY	-
*	Female pseudo-hermaphrodite	46 XX	+

* BB : Barr body.

* **SIGNS**

Goldstein's sign :

* *Cretinism and mongolism*

  ... Widened space between the great toe and adjoining toes.

Gorlin's sign :

* *Ehlers - Danlos syndrome*

  ... On asking the pt. to touch the tip of nose with the tongue he does it with ease.

Siegert's sign :

* *Mongolism*

  ... Shorttness and inward curvature of the terminal phalanges of the fifth finger

Steinberg thumb sign :

* *Marfan's syndrome*

  ... When the wrist is gripped with the opposite hand, the thumb and fifth finger overlap appreciably.

SYNDROMES

* **G deletion syndrome I (21q-) :**

  (Antimongolism syndrome)

... Partial monosomy of chromosome 21 with absence of short arm and part of long arm.

... Large ear lobes, prominent nasal bridge. Antimongoloid slant of lid fissures (eyes) and micrognathia. Mental retardation, dystrophic nails, heart disease, hypospadiasis, cryptorchidism and hypertonia.

* **G deletion syndrome II :**

  Epicanthic folds, hypotonia, syndactyly, and retarded development.

* **XX male syndrome :**

  46 XX translocation of a portion of Y chr. to X chr. (XY interchange)

... Hyalinized testes normal male, type with external and internal genitalia, gynaecomastia, shorter than normal men, increased incidence of hypospadiasis azoospermia, mean plasma testosterone is low, plasma estradiol is elevated and plasma gonodotropin levels are high.

* **Jacob's syndrome :**

  (XXX syndrome or Triple X syndrome)

  47 XXX due to nondisjunction.

... Mental retardation, microcephaly, high arched palate, abnormal dentition. Hypertelorism, epicanthus, strabismus, hypogenitalism, dysmenorrhea, amenorrhea, sterility, early onset menopause.

* **XYY syndrome :**

  47 XYY

... Growth acceleration in early or mild childhood, thick cranial vault, agenesis of frontal sinuses, myopia, thick limbs, neuromuscular incoordination and hypogonadism.

* **XYYY syndrome :**

  48 XYY

... Mental retardation, aggressive behaviour, bilaterl simian creases, Testicular abnormalities and sterility.

* Colchicine arrests cell division at the metaphase stage when the chromosomes are most suitable for study.
* Genetic information is more extensive on X chromosomes.
* Disorders related to advanced paternal age greater than 30 years include Achondroplasia; haemophilia and Marfan's syndrome.
* 1 : 300 at age 35 years old.
* 1 : 100 at age 40 years old.
* 1 : 40 at age 45 years old.
* Aging in the over of older mothers makes them more prone to non-disjunction.
* Chromosomal analysis (in growing cells) is done in late prophase.
* The most frequentsource for study of barr-bodies is desquamated cells.
* Non-specific behavioral disorders are more common than expected in multiple Y disorders.
* A reliable marker for the impending 'blast phase' in chronic myeloid leukaemia is appearance of an isochromosome for the long arm of chromosome 17.
* Polyploidy (addition of chromosomes) and Monosomy (loss of whole autosome) are lethal in man.
* All children born to XXX females have so far been reported to be normal.
* Most of the genetic enzyme deficiencies that have been elucidated are not only inherited as recessive traits but also tend to involve enzymes that participate in catabolic pathways.
* The clinical picture in autosomal recessive disorders tends to be more uniform than that of dominant diseases.
* Recessive disorders are more commonly diagnosed in children, while dominant diseases are more frequently encountered in adults.
* With recessive inheritance only one of four children in a subship is expected to be affected.
* Autosomal dominant disorders may be related to advanced paternal age effect.

* An important feature of all X-linked inheritance is the absence of male-to-male (e.e., father-to-son) transmission of the trait.
* The use of linked restriction fragment length polymorphisms (RFLPs) is important in detecting autosomal disorders before symptoms and signs are evident and in antenatal diagnosis.
* Both parents and offspring of a person homozygous for a rare recessive gene will be healthy in autosomal recessive inheritance.
* Philadelphia Chromosome (Ph1) is an acquired chromosomal abnormality associated with chronic myeloid leukaemia with 22.9 translocation.

GENETIC COUNSELING

— It is a process of communication dealing with the human problems associated with the occurrence or risk of occurrence of a genetic disorder in a family.

— The 1st step in genetic counselling is to make certain the diagnosis is correct.

Indications for genetic counseling :

1. Advanced maternal age
2. Known or suspected hereditary condition in the family
3. A foetus or child with birth defects
4. Mental retardation
5. Recurrent spontaneous abortions.
6. Exposure to known or suspected teratogens
7. Consanguinity.

Genetic counselling team :

1. The medical specialist
2. The genetic counsellor may come from a variety of backgrounds including nursing, social work, and education.
3. Additional members.

Genetic counselling facilities :

1. Teaching or University-based tertiary care hospitals.
2. Component of a specialized clinic
3. Screening programs.
4. Outreach programs

Goals of genetic counselling :

1. Comprehending the medical facts.
2. Understanding the mode of inheritance and he recurrence risks
3. Understanding the options.
4. Choosing a course of action
5. Adjusting to the condition

Counselling process :

1. Reconizing the psychologic and emotional burdens associated with the diagnosis.
   a. **Guilt** (i) Realistic guilt feelings.
   (ii) Unrealistic guilt feeling.
   b. Shame
2. Recognizing factors that affect counselling
   a. a variety of ethnic backgrounds.
   b. Socioeconomic status
3. Providing nondirective counselling
4. Helping the family relieve feelings of shame and guilt.
5. Helping the family identify its personal goals.
6. Recognizing counsellor biases.

Problems in counseling :

1. **Genetic heterogeneity** often complicates the establishment of a precise diagnosis. Similar disorders due tto mutations at different loci or involving different alleles may have different form of inheritance. **Retinitis pigmentosa** may be inherited as an autosomal **recessive** or **dominant** as well an **x-linked** condition.
2. **Phenocopies** mimic genetic disorders, are caused by environmental factors, and are, therefore, unlikely to recur. Microcephaly may have both genetic and nongenetic causes.
3. The **Sporadic case** is common in nuclear families. Here, the pedigree is not helpful, and the counsellor must depend on an accurate diagnosis. The advent of molecular methods of diagnosis has helped in some areas (eg DMD with an identified deletion) to define a recurrence risk for the family.
   Note : DMD-Duchenne muscular dystrophy
4. **Nonpaternity** or questined paternity may invalidate the risks quoted in a counselling session. Interpretation of molecular analysis is dependent upon known paternity, with the use of both direct and indirect methods. The inadvertent discovery of nonpaternity during the cause of such testing creates ethical concerns regarding whether or not to disclose the fact.

THE GENETIC CODE

First base	Second base: U	C	A	G	Third base
	Phe	Ser	Tyr	Cys	U
	Phe	Ser	Tyr	Cys	C
U	Leu	Ser	Term.	Term.	A
	Leu	Ser	Term.	Trp	G
	Leu	Pro	His	Arg	U
	Leu	Pro	His	Arg	C
C	Leu	Pro	Gln	Arg	A
	Leu	Pro	Gln	Arg	G
	Ile	Thr	Asn	Ser	U
	Ile	Thr	Asn	Ser	C
A	Ile	Thr	Lys	Arg	A
	Met (CI)	Thr	Lys	Arg	G
	Val	Ala	Asp	Gly	U
	Val	Ala	Asp	Gly	C
G	Val	Ala	Glu	Gly	A
	Val (CI)	Ala	Glu	Gly	G

Gln — glutamine, Asn — aspargine; Trp — tryptophan; Term. — nonsensory or terminator codon,

CI — Chain initiating codon.

INBORN ERRORS OF METABOLISM

A) Carbohydrate metabolism

Glycogen storage disease		*Deficiency*
Type I	von Gierke's disorder	Glucose-6-Phosphatase
Type II	Pompe's disease	a-glucosidase
Type III	Cori or Forbes disorder	Debranching enzymes
Type IV	Anderson amylopectinosis	Brancher enzyme
Type V	McArdle's disorder	Muscle phosphorylase
Type VI	Her's	Liver Phosphorylase
Type VII		Phosphofructokinase
Type VIII		Unknown
Type IX		Phosphorylase kinase
Type X		3',5-cyclic AMP dependent kinase

B) Amino acid metabolim

Disease	*Error/deficiency (def)*
Phenylkeoanuria	Phenylalanine hydroxylase deficiency
Alkaptonuria	Homogentisic acid oxidase deficiency
Homocystinuria	Cystathione synthetase def.
Cystathioninemia	Cystathionase
Hartnup disease	Decreased tryptophan
Tyrosinosis	P-hydroxy phenyl-pyruvic acid oxidase def.
Oast house disease	Methionine malabsorption
Maple Syrup Disease	Decarboxylation of ketoacids deficient
Histidinemia	Histidase def.

C) Lipid Metabolism

Disease	*Deficiency*
Fabry's disease	a-galactosidase
Gaucher's disease	Glucocerebrosidase
Niemann-Pick's disease	Sphingomyelinase
Tay Sach's disease	Hexosaminidase A
Sandhoff disease	hexosaminidase A and B
Metachromatic leukodystrophy	Arylsulfatase A
Krabbe leukodystrophy	Galactocerebrosidase

D) Mucopolysaccharidoses

Disease	*Type*	*Deficiency*
Hurler's disease	IH	a-iduronidase
Schie syndrome	IS	L-sulfoiduronate sulfatase
Hunter's disease	II	Iduronesulfate Sulphatase
Sanfilippo syndrome	IIIA	Heparan sulfate sulfamidase
Sanfilippo syndrome	IIIB	N-acetyl - a- D-glucosaminidase
Morquio syndrome	IVA	N-acetyl galactosamine-6-Phosphatase
Morquio syndrome	IVB	b-galactosidase
Maroteaxu-Lamy syndrome	VI	N-acetylgalactosimine-4-sulfatase
MPS	VII	b-glucoronidase

(e) Lipoproteinemias

Type	*Raised levels of*
I	Chylomicrons
IIa	LDL (b type)
IIb	LDL and VLDL (b) (pre-b)
III	Mostly LDL and some VLDL
IV	VLDL (Pre-b)
V	Chylomicrons and VLDL

* LDL is rish in cholesterol and type V is secondary to diabetes mellitus

(f) ***Miscellaneus***

Disease	*Defect*
Galactosemia	Galactose-1-phosphate Uridyl transferase deficiency
Albinism	Tyrosinase deficiency
Lesch-Nyhan syndrome	Hypoxanthine Guanine phosphoribosyl transferase deficiency
Refsum's disease	Phytic acid malabsorption
Gout	Purine metabolism disturbed
Orotic aciduria	Pyrimidine disturbed

COMPARISION OF NUCLEIC ACIDS

RNA	*DNA*
a. Built up from Adenine and guanine, cytosine and uracil, with ribose and phosphoric acid.	a. Built up from Adenine and guanine, cytosine and thymine, with deoxyribose and phosphoric acid.
b. Present in cell cytoplasm and nucleolus.	b. Present in Nucleus, probably in the chromosomes.
c. Carries no "genetic information" and undergoes no mutation.	c. Carries "genetic information" from one generation of cells to the next and undergoes mutation.
d. Concerned with protein synthesis.	d. Concerned with protein synthesis.
e. Contains 60 to 6000 nucleotides, molecules are unbranched, structure is less rigid.	e. Contains 1600 to 9000 nucleotides, molecules are long and thread like having a length of about 250 times greater than their breadth, structure is highly complex.

EXAMPLES OF AUTOSOMAL ABNORMALITIES ASSOCIATED WITH RECOGNISED CLINICAL SYNDROMES

Chromosome abnormality	*Syndrome*	*Clinical features*
Trisomy-21 Translocation 13-15/21 Translocation 22/21 Translocation 21/21	Down's	Characteristic facies Mental retardation Hypotonia Congenital heart disease Simian palmar crease
Trisomy-13	Patau's	Motor and mental retardation Microcephaly Microphthalmia Cleft palate/hare lip Polydactyly Congenital heart disease

Trisomy-18	Edwards	Motor and mental retardation Flexation deformities of fingers Micrognathia 'Rocker-bottom' feet Congenital heart disease
4p- Wolf's		Mental retardation Abnormal facies Cleft palate Coloboma Epilepsy Hypospadias Scalp defects
5p-	Cri du chat	Mental retardation Microcephaly Hypertelorism Characteristic cry

CLINICAL FEATURES OF KLINEFELTER'S AND TURNER'S SYNDROME

Klinefelter's Syndrome	*Turner's Syndrome*
Sterility	Primary amenorrhoea
Small testes	Sterility
Euncuchoid body proportions	Lack of secondary sexual characteristics
Gynaecomastia	Short stature
Mental retardation	Various congenital abnormalities (note coarctation of the aorta)

PARTIAL LIST OF HUMAN GENETIC DISEASES THAT HAVE BEEN MAPPED TO SPECIFIC CHROMOSOMES

Chromosome	*Disease*
1	Elliptocytosis
	Rh erythroblastosis
	Porphyria cutanea tarda
2.	Protein C deficiency
3	Protein S deficiency
	Orotic aciduria
4	Huntington's disease

5	Gardner syndrome
	Familial polyposis coli
6	Hemochromatoosis
	Congenital adrenal hyperplasia (21-hydroxylase deficiency)
7	Cystic fibrosis
	Ehlers-Danlos syndrome (one form)
	Osteogenesis imperfecta (one form)
8.	None found
9	Galactosemia
	Nail-patella syndrome
10	Multiple endocrine neoplasia type 2
11	Syndrome of Wilms' tumor, aniridia, gonado-blastoma, retardation,
	β-Thalassemia
	Sickle cell anemia
12	Phenylketonuria
	von Willebrand's disease
13	Retinoblastoma
	Wilson's disease
14	Nucleoside diphosphorylase deficiency (immunodeficiency)
15	Prader-Willi syndrome
	Tay-Sachs disease
16	α-Thalassemia
	Gout due to adenine phosphoribosyl transferase deficiency
	LCAT deficiency
17	Growth hormone deficiency (type A)
	von Recklinghausen neurofibromatosis
19	Familial hypercholesterolesterolemia
	Familial type 3 hyperlipoproteinemia
	Myotonic dystrophy
	Complement C3 deficiency
20	Adenosine deaminase deficiency
	(immuno deficiency)
21	Alzheimer's disease
	Homocystinuria
22	Metachromatic leukodystrophy
	Hurler syndrome (mucopolysaccharidoses I)
	Scheie's syndrome (mucopolysaccharidoses V)

X	X-linked ichthyosis due to placental steroid sulfantase deficiency
	Ocular albinism
	Chronic granulomatous disease
	Duchenne muscular dystrophy
	Testicular feminization syndrome
	Phosphoglycerate kinase deficiency (hemolytic anemia)
	Fabry's disease
	Lesch-Nyhan syndrome
	Fragile site associated with X-linked mental retardation
	Colour blindness
	Hemophilia A
	Glucose-6-phosphate dehydrogenase (G6PD) deficiency

HLA ANTIGENS AND DISEASE, SHOWING THE MOST HIGHLY ASSOCIATED ANTIGENS

Disease	*Antigen*
RHEUMATIC	
Ankylosing spondylitis	B27
Reiter's syndrome	B27
Acute anterior uveitis	B27
Reactive arthritis (yersinia, salmonella, goonococcus)	B27
Psoriatic arthritis, central	B27 Bw 38
Psoriatic arthritis, peripheral	B27 Bw38
Juvenile rheumatoid, arthritis	B27 DRw8
Juvenile arthritis, pauciarticular	DR5
Rheumatoid arthritis	Dw 4/DR4
Sjogren's syndrome	Dw3
Systemic lupus erythematosus	DR3
Systemic lupus erythematosus	DR4
GASTROINTESTINAL	
Gluten-sensitive enteropathy	DR3
Chronic active hepatitis	DR3
Ulcerative colitis	B5

HEMATOLOGIC	
Idiopathic hemochromatosis	A3
	B14
	A3, B14
Pernicious anemia	DR5
SKIN	
Dermatitis herpetiformis	Dw3
Psoriasis vulgaris	Cw6
Psoriasis vulgaris (Japanese)	Cw6
Pemphigus vulgaris (Jews)	DR4
	A10
Behcet's disease	B5
ENDOCRINE	
Type 1 diabetes mellitus	DR4
	DR3
	DR2
	BfF1
Hyperthyroidism	B8
	Dw3
Co Hyperthyroidism (Japanese)	Bw35
Adrenal insufficiency	Dw3
Subacute thyroiditis (de Quervain)	Bw35
Hashimoto's thyroiditis	DR5
Congenital adrenal hyperplasia	Bw 47
NEUROLOGIC	
Myasthenia gravis	B8
	DR3
Multiple sclerosis	DR2
Manic-depressive disorder	Bw16
Narcolepsy	DR2
Schizophrenia	A28
RENAL	
Idiopathic membranous glomerulonephritis	DR3
Goodpasture's syndrome (anti-GBM)	DR2
Minimal change disease (steroid response)	B12
Polycystic kidney disease	B5
IgA nephropathy	DR4
Gold nephropathy	DR3
	DR4

INFECTIOUS	
Tuberculoid leprosy (Asians)	B8
Paralytic polio	Bw 16
Low vs. high response to vaccinia virus	Cw 3
IMMUNODEFICIENCY	
IgA deficiency (blood donors)	DR3

PEDIGREE CHARACTERISTICS OF AUTOSOMAL DOMINANT DISORDERS

1. Each affected individual has an affected parent, unless the condition arose by fresh mutation in the given individual (Because of wide variability in severity of dominant traits, the parent may be too mildly affected to be recognized as a case)
2. An affected individual and a normal mate will have, on the average, affected and normal children in equal proportions.
3. Normal children of an affected person will have all normal offspring.
4. Males and females are affected in equal proportions.
5. Affected males and females are equally likely to transmit the condition to male and female offspring. Specifically, male-to-male transmission occurs.
6. Homozygotes may be born if two affected persons (heterozygotes) marry. Homozygotes are usually more severely affected than heterozygotes.
7. On the average, the age of fathers of sporadic (new mutation) cases is elevated.
8. The more severely the disorder interferes with reproduction, the larger is the proportion of cases that are sporadic ("new mutations").

PEDIGREE CHARACTERISTICS OF AUTOSOMAL RECESSIVE DISORDERS

1. The parents are usually clinically normal.
2. The larger the family, the more often will more than one child be affected.
3. The rarer the mutant gene in the population, the more often will the parents be related.

4. In marriages between individuals, each with the same recessive disease, all their offspring will be affected.
5. Affected individuals who marry normal individuals have only normal offspring (unless the normal spouse is a carrier).
6. The sexes are affected in equal proportions
7. If an affected individual marries a heterozygote, as is more likely to occur with consanguineous marriage, half the children would be affected, and a pedigree pattern simulating dominant inheritance would result.

PEDIGREE CHARACTERISTICS OF SEX LINKED (X-LINKED) RECESSIVE DISORDERS.

A. When the disorder is such that affected males do not reproduce (e.g. Duchenne muscular dystrophy, testicualr feminization syndrome, etc.)
   1. Only males are affected
   2. About two-thirds of cases have a carrier mother from whom the mutation in the X chromosome from the mother
   3. In the inherited form, affected males may have affected brothers and affected maternal uncles. The new mutation cases are sporadic, i.e, isolated cases
   4. The sisters of inherited cases have a 50 percent chance of being carriers for the gene
   5. A carrier sister transmits the gene to half her sons, who are affected, and to half her daughters, who are carriers.
   6. Unaffected do not transmit the disorder.

B. When the disorder is such that affected males may reproduce (e.g. hemophilias A and B, G6PD deficiency, etc.)
   1. The proportion of cases that are inherited rises further above two-thirds, the less is the reduction of average number of children produced by affected males.
   2. Affected males transmit the gene to all their daughters and to none of their sons
   3. All phenotypically normal daughters of affected males are carriers
   4. If married to a carrier female, affected males will have daugh ters, half of whom are homozygous and affected, half of whom are normal but carriers.
   5. Rare heteozygous females may be affected ("manifesting heterozygotes"), because of chances of lyonization.

PEDIGREE CHARACTERISTICS OF X-LINKED DOMINANT DISORDERS

1. Both males and females are affected, but females tend to be affected about twice as often as males
2. An affected female transmits the disorder to half her sons and half her daughters, on the average.
3. An affected male transmits the disorder to all his daughters and to none of the sons.
4. On the average, the heterozygous affected female tends to be less severelly affected than the hemizygous male, and the disorder is more variable in females.

DIFFERENTIAL DIAGNOSIS OF SHORT STATURE

		Constitutional delay in growth	*Familial short stature*	*Pituitary dwarfism*	*Hypothyroidism*	*Turner syndrome*
1.	Family history	+ve	+ve	usually-ve	-ve	usually-ve
2.	Birth weight & height	N	↓	N	N	Slightly reduced
3.	Pattern of growth birth	Slow from birth months after birth	Slow from birth	Slow from a few	Slow from	Slow from birth
4.	Epiphyseal development	moderate but not progressive	almost normal	progressive retardation	marked retardation	within normla with variation
5.	Clinical features normal	immaute, later	mature	immature	infantile facies	characteristic
	Puberty	delayed	normal	delayed	delayed	usualy no signs
	Serum cholesterol	N	N	↑	↑	N
	hGH cholesterol	N	N	↓	N	N
	Gonadotrophin levels (after puberty)	N	N	↓ except in isolated hGH deficiency	N (or ↑)	↑

COMMON ABNORMALITIES IN DOWN'S SYNDROME

Neonatal

Hypotonia, Lax joints and absent Moro reflex

Excess nuchal skin and 'well behaved'

Craniofacial

Brachycephaly and epicanthic folds

Upward slanting palpebral fissures

Brushifield spots in iris

Small ears and protruding tongue

Limbs

Small middle phalanx of fifth finger

Single palmar crease

High incidence of ulnar loops on fingers

Wide gap and plantar crease between first and second toes

Cardiac

Common atrioventricular canal

Atrial septal defect and ventricular septal defect

Patent ductus arteriosus Tetralogy of Fallot

Other

Short stature and strabismus

Duodenal atresia and anal atresia

Increased incidence of leukaemia and thyroid disororders

RISK OF DOWN'S SYNDROME IN RELATION TO MATERNAL AGE.*

Maternal age at delivery (years)	*Incidence of Down's syndrome in liveborn infants*
30	1 in 700
35	1 in 450
36	1 in 400
37	1 in 250
38	1 in 200
39	1 in 150
40	1 in 100
41	1 in 80
42	1 in 60
43	1 in 50
44	1 in 40
45	1 in 30

* The maternal age-specific risk of Down's syndrome tends to be higher in chorion villous biopsy and amniocentesis studies. Presumably this reflects preferential spontaneous loss of Down's syndrome conceptions throughout pregnancy.

CLINICAL FEATURES OF TRISOMY 18.

Craniofacial

Prominent occiput
Low set dysplastic ears
Narrow short palpebral fissures
Small mouth and micrognathia

Limbs

Clenched hands and overlapping fingers
Hypoplastic nails
Rocker bottom feet and talipes
Short dorsiflexed big toes

Cardiac

Ventricular and atrial septal defects
Patent ductus arteriosus
Coarctation of aorta
Bicuspid aortic valve

Other

Hypoplastic radlii
Tracheo-oesophageal fistula
Oesophageal atresia
Short sternum
Cryptorchidism
Renal anomalies
Spina bifida

COMMON CLINICAL FINDINGS IN TRISOMY 13.

Craniofacial

Microcephaly
Facies type I, holoprosencephaly and hypotelorism
Cyclops, absent philtrum and nares
Facies type II, microphthalmia and large bulbous nose
Cleft lip and plate
Small auricles, often low set
Occipital scalp defects

Limbs

Single palmar crease
Post-axial polydactyly
Hyperconvex nails

Cardiac

Atrial and ventricular septal defects
Patent ductus arteriosus and dextrocardia

Other

Single umbilical artery
Cryptorchidism
Exomphalos
Polycystic kidneys

CLINICAL FEATURES OF TURNER'S SYNDROME.

Hallmarks

Short stature and ovarian dysgenesis

Craniofacial

Prominent ears
Neck webbing
Low posterior hairline
Ptosis

Limbs

Cubitus valgus
Short fourth metacarpal
Puffy hands and feet
Hyperconvex nails

Other

Coarctation of aorta
Horseshoe kidney
Shield chest
Madelung deformity
Conductive deafness (mild)

EXAMPLES OF AUTOSOMAL DOMINANT DISORDERS

System	*Principal clinial features*
Skeletal and connective tissue	
Achondroplasia	Large head, short stature and short limbs
Marfan's syndrome	Tall stature, lens dislocation and aortic aneurysm
Osteogenesis imperfecta	Brittle bones, blue sclerac and deafness
Malformations	

Apert's syndrome	Craniosynostosis and syndactyly
Holt-Oram syndrome	Atrial septal defect and thumb abnormality
Noonan's syndrome	Pulmonary stenosis, ptosis and neck webbing
Phakomatosis	
Neurofibromatosis	Cafe-au-lait patches and neurofibromata
Tuberous sclerosis	Adenoma sebaceum and depigmented naevi
Neurological	
Huntington's chorea	Adult onset chorea and dementia
Myotonic dystrophy	Myotonia, muscle weakness and wasting
Peroneal muscular atrophy	Distal muscle weakness and wasting
Gastrointestinal	
Peutz-Jeghers syndrome	Oral freckling and intestinal polyps
Polyposis coli	Intestinal polyps, and high risk of malignancy
Haematological and metabolic	
Familial hypercholesterolaemia	Xanthomata and coronary artery disease
Spherocytosis	Mild haemolysis
Von Willebrand's disease	Haemorrhage and factor VIII deficiency
Renal	
Adult polycystic kidney disease	Renal cysts and renal failure
Alport's syndrome (some forms)	Nephritis and deafness

AUTOSOMAL RECESSIVE DISORDERS SHOWING HIGH INCIDENCE IN PARTICULAR ETHNIC GTOUPS

Ethnic grouo	*Disorder*
Afro - Carribeans	Sickle cell disease
Ashkenazi Jews	Familial dysautonomia
	Tay Sach's disease
Caucasian	Cystic fibrosis
Eskimos	Congenital adrenal hyperplasia
Finns	Congenital nephrosis
Greek - Cypriots	β thalassaemia
Norwegians	α –1 antitrypsin deficiency

CLICNICAL FEATURES AND EXAMPLES OF X - LINKED DISORDERS

Reccessive	
Red - green colour blindness	Mildly impaired colour vision
G-6-PD deficiency	Drug-induced haemolysis
Haemophilia A	Haemorrhage, factor VIII deficiency
Haemophilia B (Christmas disease)	Haemorrhage, factor IX deficiency
Bruton's agammaglobulinacmia	Recurrent bacterial infection
Duchenne muscular dystrophy	Progressive muscle weakness, pseudohypertrophy
Lesch-Nyhan syndrome	Neurodegeneration, self -mutilation
Dominant	
Pseudohypoparathyroidism	Short stature, obesity, cataracts
Vitamin D-resistant rickets,	Rickets, low serum phosphate
Dominant	
Incontinentia pigmenti	Abnormalities of teeth, eyes and skin pigmentation; lethal in males

CRITERIA FOR THE DIAGNOSIS OF MARFAN'S SYDNROME

Major criteria	*Minor criteria*
Mitral incompetence	
Arachnodactyly	
with floppy valve	High arched palate
Aortic incompetence	Funnel chest
Dilated aortic root	Asthenic build
Dissecting aortic aneurysm	Joint laxity (especially ankles)
	Flat feet
Dislocation of the lens	Scoliosis
Trembling iris	Spontaneous pneumothorax
	Floppy mitral valve without incompetence
	Severe myopia (.4 dioptres)

INDICATIONS FOR CYTOGENETIC ANALYSIS.

1. Patients with malformations suggestive of one of the recorgnized syndromes associated with a specific chromosome aberration.
2. Patients of any age who are grossly retarded physically or mentally, especially if there are associated anomalies.

3. Any patient with ambiguous internal or external genitalia or suspected hermaphroditism.
4. Girls with primary amenorrhea and boys with delayed pubertal development. Up to 25% of patients with primary amenorrhea have a chromosomal abnormality.
5. Males with learning or behavioural disorders who are taller than expected (based on parental height).
6. Certain malignant and premalignant diseases
7. Parents of a patient with chromosome translocation.
8. Parents of a patient with a suspected chromosomal syndrome if there is a family history of similarly affected children.
9. Couples with a history of multiple spontaneous abortions of unknown cause.
10. Couples who are infertile after more comon obstetric and urologic causes have been excluded.
11. Prenatal diagnosis

EMPIRIC RISKS FOR SOME CONGENITAL DISORDERS.

Mental deficiency of unknown cause : Incidence 3:1000

Risks for siblings

Both parents norma: l 5-13% retarded.

One parent retarded : 20% retarded

Both parents retarded : 42% retarded

Anencephaly and spina bifida : Incidence (average) 1: 1000

One affected child :2-3%

Two affected children : 10-12%

One affected parent :2-3%

Hydrocephalus : Incidence 1:2000 newborns

Occasional X-linked recessive

Often associated with neural tube defect

Some environmental etiologies, eg, toxoplasmosis

Recurrence risk, one affected child

Hydrocephalus : 1%

Some CNS abnormality : 3%

Cleft Lip and/or palate : Incidence (average) 1:1000

One affected child : 2-4%

One affected parent : 2-4%

Two affected children : 10%

One affected parent, one affected child : 10-20-%

Cleft palate : Incidence 1:2000

One affected child : 2%

Two affected children : 6-8%

One affected parent : 4-6%

One affected parent, one affected child : 15-20%

Congenital heart disease : Incidence 8:1000

One affected child : 2-3%

One affected parent, one affected child : 10%

Clubfoot: Incidence 1:1000 (male-female=2.1)

One affected child :2-3%

Congenital dislocated hip : Incidence 1:1000 (female>male) with marked regional variation

One child affected : 2-14%

Pyloric stenosis : Incidence, males : 1:200; females : 1:1000

Male index patient

Brothers	3.2%
Sons	6.8%
Sisters	3.0%
Daughters	1.2%

Female index patient

Brothers	13.2%
Sons	20.5%
Sisters	2.5%
Daughters	11.1%

CURRENTLY RECOGNIZED CONTIGUOUS GENE SYNDROMES

Syndrome	Abnormal Chromosome Segment
Prader-Willi syndrome	del 15q11
DiGeorge syndrome	del 22q11
Langer-Gideon syndrome	del 8q24
Miller-Dicker syndrome	del17p13
Retinoblastoma/mental retardation	del 13q14
Beckwith-Wiedemann syndrome	del 11p15
Wilms tumor with aniridia, genitourinary malformations, and mental retardation	del 11p13

CLINICAL PHENOTYPES RESULTING FROM ANEUPLOIDY

Condition	Karyotype	Incidence at Birth
Trisomy 13	47, XX or XY, +13	1:15,000
Trisomy 18	47, XX or XY, +18	1:11,000
Trisomy 21 (Down's syndrome)	47, XX or XY, +21	1:900
Klinefelter's syndrome	47,XXY	1:1000 males
XYY	47, XYY	1:1000 males
Turner's syndrome	45,X	1:7500 females
XXX syndrome	47, XXX	1:1000 females

REPRSENTATIVE INBORN ERRORS OF METABOLISM.

General Class of Defect	Examples	Biochemical Defect	Inheritance[1]
Aminoacidopathy	Phenylketonuria	Phenylalanine hydroxylase	AR
Connective tissue	Osteogenesis imperfecta type II	α1(I) and α2 (I) procollagen	AD
Gangliosidosis	Tay-Sachs disease	Hexosaminidase A	AR
Glycogen storage disease	Type 1	Glucose-6-phosphatase	AR
Immune function	Chronic granulomatous disease	Cytochrome b,β chain	XL

Lipid metabolism	Familial hypecholesterolemia	LDL receptor	AD
Mucopolysaccharidosis	MPS II (Hunter's syndrome)	Iduronate sulfatase	XL
Porphyria	Acute intermittent	Porphobilinogen deaminaase	AD
Transport	Cystic fibrosis	CF transmembrane conductance regular	AR

[1]AR = Autosomal recessive; AD=autosomal dominant; XL=X-linked recessive.

REQUIREMENTS FOR EFFECTIVE SCREENING FOR INBORN ERRORS OF METABOLISM.

1. The disease should be clinically severe or have potentially severe consequences.
2. The natural history of the disease should be understood.
3. Effective treatment should be generally available and depend on early diagnosis for optimal results.
4. The disease incidence should be high enough to warrant screening.
5. The screening test should have favourable specificity (low false-positive rate) and sensitivity (low false-negative rate).
6. The screening test should be available for and used by the entire population at risk.
7. An adequate system for follow-up of positive results should be provided.
8. The economic cost-benefit analysis should favor screening and treatment.

MANNER OF PRESENTATION OF INBORN ERRORS OF METABOLISM.

Presentation and Course	Examples
Acute metabolic disease of the neonate	Galactosemia, urea cycle disorders
Chronic disorders with little progression	Phenylketonuria, hypothyroidism
Chronic disorders with insidious, incessant progression	Tay-Sachs disease
Disorders causing abnormaliteis of structure	Skeletal dysplasias, Marfan's syndrome
Disorders of transport	Cystinuria, lactase deficiency
Disorder that determine susceptibilities	LDL receptor deficiency, agammaglobulinemia
Episodic disorders	Most porphyrias, G6PD deficiency
Disorders causing anemia	Pyruvate kinase deficiency, hereditary spherocytosis
Disorders interfering hemostasis	Hemophilia A and B, von Willebrand disease
Congenital disorders with no psssibility of reversal	Testicular feminization
Disorders with protein manifestations	Pseudohyparathyroidism, hereditary amyloidoses
Inborn errors with no clinical effects	Pentosuria, histidinemia

SELECTED DNA PROBES WITH CURRENT DIAGNOSTIC APPLICATIONS.

Gene Probe	Disorder	Diagnostic Application
β-globin	Sickle cell disease	Prenatal screening
	Beta thalassemia	Prenatal screening
αGlobin	Alpha thalassemia	Prenatal screening
	Polycystic kidney disease	Presymptomatic, prenatal screening
Factor VIII	Hemophiia A	Prenatal screening carrier detection
Dystrophin	Duchenne's muscular dystrophy	Presymptomatic, Prenatal screening, carier detection
α-AP	α1-Antiprotease deficiency	Prenatal screening
Para hydroxylase	Phenylketonuria	Prenatal screening
CFTR	Cystic fibrosis	Prenatal, presymptomatic screening, carrier detection
Ternucleotide repeat (CAG) in Huntingtion	Huntington's disease	Presymptomatic, Prenatal screening
Growth hormone	Growth hormone deficiency	Prenatal screening, carrier detection, early diagnosis
CXR	Hemochromatosis	Presymptomatic, Prenatal screening

CHROMOSOME ABERRATIONS ASSOCITED WITH REPRESENTATIVE SOLID TUMORS

Tumor	Chromosome Aberration
Meningioma	del(22)(111)1
Neuroblastoma	del(1)(p36) or amplification
Renal cell carcinoma	del(3)(p-14.2-p25) or translocation of this region
Retinoblastoma, osteosarcoma	del (13)(q14.1) or translocation of this region
Small-cell lung carcinoma	del(3)(p-14-p23)
Wilm's tumor	del(11)(p15)

Nomenclature means, "a deletion at band q11 of chromosome 22*.

CHROMOSOMAL ABERRATIONS ASSOCIATED WITH REPRESENTATIVE HEMATOLOGIC MALIGNANCIES.

Tumor	Chromosomal Aberration
Leukemias	
Acute m' eloblastic	t(8;21) (q22;q11)1
Acute p:omyelocytic	t(15;17) (122;q11-q12)
Acute monocytic	t(10;11)(p15-o11;q23)
Chronic myelogenous	t(8;22)(q23;q11)
Lymphomas	
Burkitt's	t(8;14)(q24.1;q32.3)
B cell	t(1;14)(q42;q43)
T cell	inv, del, and 1 of 1p13-p12
Premalignancy	
Polycythemia vera	del(20)(q11)

[1]Nomenclature means, "a translocation with the union at band q22 of chromosome 8 and q11 of chromosome 21."

SOME OF THE "UNSAFE" AND "PROBABLY SAFE" DRUGS USED IN THE TREATMENT OF ACUTE PORPHYRIAS

Unsafe	Probably Safe
Alcohol	Acetaminophen
Alkylating agents	Amitryptyline
Barbiturates	Aspirin
Carbamazepine	Atropine
Chlorpropramide	Beta-adrenergic blockers
Cloroquine	Chloral hydrate
Clonidine	Chlordiazepoxide
Dapsone	Diazepam
Ergots	Digoxin
Erythromycin	Diphenyhydramine
Estrogens, synthetic	Guanethidine
Food addictives	Glucocorticoids

Glutethimide
Griseofulvin
Hydralazine
Ketamine
Meprobamate
Methyldopa
Metoclopramide
Nortriptyline
Pentazocine
Phenytoin
Progestins
Pyrazinamide
Rifampin
Spironolactone
Succinimides
Sulfonamides
Theophylline
Tolazamide
Tolbutamide
Valproic acid
Hyoscine
Ibuprofen
Imipramine
Insulin
Lithium
Naproxen
Nitrofurantoin
Opioid analgesics
Penicillamine
Penicillin and derivatives
Phenothiazines
Procaine
Streptomycin
Succinylcholine
Tetracycline
Thiouracil

SELECTED DATABASES RELEVANT FOR GENOMICS AND GENETIC DISORDERS

Site	URL	Comment
National Center for Biotechnology Information (NCBI)	http://www.ncbi.nim.nih.gov/ computational biology	Molecular biology information, public database. Software for analyzing genome data Extensive links to other databases, genome resources, and educational primers
National Human Genome Research Institute	http://www.genome.gov/	Web links providing information about the human genome sequence, genomes of other organisms, and genomic research
Ensembl Genome browser Man (OMIM)	http://www.ncbi.nim.nih.gov/omim/	Online compendium of Mendelian disorders and human genes causing genetic disorders
Office of Biotechnology Activities National Insititutes of Health	www4.od.nih.gov/oba/	Information about recombinant DNA and gene transfer Medical ethical, legal, and social issue raised by genetic testing Medical, ethical, legal, and social issue raised by xenotransplantation

SELECTED DATABASES RELEVANT FOR GENOMICS AND GENETIC DISORDERS

Site	URL	Comment
American College of Medical Genetics	http://www.acmg.net/	Extensive links to other diatabases relevant for the diagnosis, treatment and prevention of genetic disease.
Cancer Genome Anatomy Project (CGAP)		http://cgap.nci.nih.gov/ Information about gene expression profiles of normal, precancer, and cancer cells
Gen Link	http://www.genlink.wustl.edu	Multimedia database resource for human genetics and telomere research
Gene Test-GeneClinics	http://www.genetests.org/	International directory of genetic testing laboratories and prenatal diagnosis clinics Reviews and educational materials
Dolan DNA Learning Center, Cold Spring Harbor Laboratories	http://www.dnalc.org	Reviews and educatinal materials disorders, DNA, eugenics, and genetic origin
HUGO Gene Nomenclature	http://www.gene.ucl.ac.uk/nomenclature	Gene names and symbols
MITOMAP, a human mitochondrial genome database	http://www.mitomap.org	A compendium of polymorphisms and mutations of the human mitochondrial DNA
Mitochondrial disorders	http://www.neuro.wustl.edu/neuromuscular/mitosyn.html	Overview on clinical syndromes associated with mtDNA mutations.
DNA repeat sequences & disease	http://www.neuro.wustl.edu/neuromuscular/mother/dnarep.htm	Overview on clinical syndromes associated with DNA repeats
Online Mendelian Inheritance in Animals (OMIA)	http://www.angis.su.oz.au/Databases/BIRX/omia	Online compendium of Mendelian disorders in animals
The Jackson Laboratory	http://www.jax.org/	Information about murine models and the mouse genome

SELECTED EXAMPLES OF DISEASES CAUSED BY MUTATIONS AND REARRANGEMENTS IN TRANSCRIPTIN FACTOR CLASSES

Transcription Factor Class	Example	Associated Disorder
Nuclear receptors	Androgen receptor	Complete or partial androgen insensitivity (recessive missense mutations). Spinobulbar muscular atrophy (CAG repeat expansion)
Zinc finger proteins	WT-1	WAGR syndrome: Wilm's tumor, aniridia, genitourinary malformations, mental retardation
Basic helix-loop-helix	MITF	Waardenburg syndrome type 2 A
Homeobox	IPF1	Maturity onset of diabetes mellitus type 4 (heterozygous mutation/haploinsufficiency) Pancreatic agenesis (homozygous mutation)
Leucine zipper	Retina leucine zipper (NRL)	Autosomal dominant retinitis pigmentosa

High-mobility group (HMG) proteins	SRY	Sex-reversal
Forkhead	HNF4α HNF1α, HNF1β	Maturity-onset of diabetes mellitus types 1,3,5
Paired box	PAX-3	Waardenburg syndrome types 1 and 3
T-box	TBX-5	Holt-Oram syndrome (thumb anomalies, atrial or ventricular septum defects, phocomelia)
Cell cycle control proteins	P53	Li-Fraumeni syndrome, other cancers
Coactivators	CREB binding protein (CBP)	Rubenstein-Taybi syndrome
General transcription	TATA-binding protein (TBP)	Spinocerebellar ataxia 17 (CAG expansion)
Transcription elongation	VHL	von Hippel-Lindau syndrome (renal cell carcinoma, pheochromocytoma, pancreatic tumors, hemangioblastomas) Autosomal dominant inheritance, somatic inactivation of second allele
Runt	CBFA2	Familial thrombocytopenia with propensity to acute myelogenous leukemia
Chimeric proteins due to translocations	PML-RAR	Acute promyelocytic leukemia t(15;17) (q22;q11.212) translocation

GENETIC MODIFIED ANIMALS

Commonly Used Description	Technical Principle	Remarks
Transgenic	Pronuclear infection of transgene	Commonly used Geonomic DNA or cNDA constructs Random integration of transgene Variable copy numbers of transgene Variable expression in each individual founder Gain of functionmodels due to overexpression using tissue-specific promoters Loss of function models using antisense and dominat negative transgenes Inducible expression possible (Tetracycline, ecdysone) Applicable to severe species

(Targeted) Knockout	Substitutin of functional gne with inactive gene by homologous recombination in embryonic stem cells	Predominantly used in mice Tissue specific knockout possible (Cre/lox) Absence of phenotype possible due to redundancy
(Targeted) Knockin	Introductino of subtle mutation(s) into gene by substitution of endogenous gene with gene carrying a specific mutation. Homologous recombination in embryonic stem cells	Predominantly used in mice Can accurately model human disease
Forward genetics	Mutations created randomly by ENU (N-ethyl-N-nitrourea)	Selection of phenotype followed by genetic characterization Useful for cloning of novel genes
Cloning	Introduction of nucleus into enucleated eggs (nuclear transfer)	Successful in several mammalian species including sheep (Dolly), mice, cows, monkeys Cloning of genetically identical individuals May affect life span Ethical concerns

SELECTED TRINUCLEOTIDE REPEAT DISORDER

Disease	Locus	Repeat	Triplet Length Nomral/Disease	Inheritance	Gene Product
X-Chromosomal spinobulbar muscular atrophy (SBMA)	Xq11-q12	CAG	11-34/40-62	XR	Androgen receptor
Fragile X-syndrome (FRAXA)	Xq27.3	CGG	6-50/200-300	XR	FMR-protein
Fragile X-syndrome (FRAXE)	Xq28	GCC	6-25/>200	XR	FMR-2 protein
Dystrophia myotonica (DM)	19q13.2-q13.3	CTG	5-30/200-1000	AD, variable penetrance	Myotonin protein kinase
Huntington disease (HD)	4p16.3	CAG	11-34/37-121	AD	Huntington
Spinocerebellar ataxiay type 1 (SCA1)	6p21.3-21.2	CAG	19-36/39-83	AD	Ataxin 1
Spinocerebellar ataxia type type 2 (SCA2)	12q24.1	CAG	15-31/34-400	AD	Ataxin 2
Spinocerebellar ataxia type 3 (SCA3); Machado Joseph disease (MD)	14q21	CAG	13-36/55-86	AD	SC3/MJD1
Spinocerebellar ataxia type 6 (SCA6, CACNAIA)	19p13.1-13.2	CAG	4-16/20-33	AD	Alpha 1A voltage-dependent calcium channel
Spinocerebellar ataxia type 7 (SCA7)	3p21.1-p12	CAG	4-19/37 •300	AD	Ataxin 7
Spinocerebellar ataxia type 12 (SCA12)	5q31	CAG	6-26/66-78	AD	Protein phosphatase 2A
Dentorubral pallidoluysiane atrophy (DRPLA)	12q	CAG	7-23/49-75	AD	Atrophin
Friedreich ataxia (FRDA1)	9q13-21	GAA	7-22/200-900	AR	Frataxin

SELECTED EXAMPLES OF LOCUS HETEROGENEITY

Phenotype	Gene	Chromosomal Location	Protein
Familial hypertrophic cardiomyopathy			
Genes encoding for sarcomeric proteins	MYH7	14q12	Myosin heavy chain beta
	TNNT2	1q2	Troponin-T2
	TPM1	15q22.1	Tropomyosin α
	MYBPC3	11p11q	Myosin binding protein C
	TNN13	19q13.4	Troponin 1
	MYL3	3p	Myosin light chain 3
	MYL2	12q23-24.3	Myosin light chain 2
	TTN	2q24.3	Cardiac titin
	ACTC	15q11	Cardiac alpha actin
	MYH6	14q1	Myosin heavy chain alpha
	TNNC1	3p21.3-3p14.3	Cardiac troponin C
Nonsarcomeric proteins	MTT1	Mitochondrial	tRNA isoleucine and tRNA glycine
	PRKAG2	7q35q36	AMP-activiated protein kinase γ2 subunit
	DMPK	19q13	Myotonin protein kiase (myotonic dystrophy)
	FRDA	9q13	Frataxin (Friedreich ataxia)
Polycystic kidney disease			
	PKD1	16q13.3-1312	Polycystin 1 (AD) :
	PKD2	4q21-23	Polycystin 2(AD)
	PKHD1	6p21.1-p12	Fibrocystin (AR)
Familial breast cancer			
BRCA1	BRCA1	17q21	BRCA1 (RNA polymerase II component)
BRCA2	BRCA2	13q12.3	BRCA2

SELECTED MITOCHONDRIAL DISEASES

Disease/Syndrome	MIM#
MELAS syndrome : mitochondrial myopathy with encephalopathy, lactic acidosis, and stroke	540000 540050
Leber's optic atrophy : hereditary optical neuropathy	535000
Kearns-Sayre syndrome (KSS): ophthalmoplegia, pigmental degeneration of the retina, cardiomyopathy	530000
MERPF syndrome: myoclonic epilepsy and ragged red fibers	545030
Maternally inherited myopathy and cardiomyopathy (MMC)	590050
Neurogenic muscular weakness with ataxia and retinitis pigmentosa (NARP)	258470
Pearson syndrome (PEAR): bone marrow and pancreatic failure	557000
Autosomal dominant inherited mitochondrial myopathy with mitochondrial deletion (admimy)	157640
Somatic mutations in cytochrome bgene: exercise intolerance, lactic acidosis, complex III deficiency, muscle pain, ragged-red fibers	

GENETIC APPROACHES FOR IDENTIFYING DISEASE GENES

Method	Indications and Advantages	Limitations
Linkage analysis	Analysis of monogenic traits Suitable for genome scan Control population not required Useful for multifactorial disorders in isolated populations	Difficult to collect large informative pedigrees Difficult to obtain sufficient statistical power for complex traits
Allele-sharing methods		
Affected sib and relative pair analyses	Suitable for identification of susceptibility gens in polygenic and multifactorial disorders	Difficult to collect sufficient number of subject Difficult to obtain sufficient
Sib pair analysis	Control population not required if allele frequencies are known Statistical power can be increasd by including parents and relatives	
Association studies		
Case-control studies Linkage disequilibrium Transmission distortion test	Suitable for identification of susceptibility genes in polygenic and multifactorial disorders variants of known candidate loc Does not necessarily need relatives	Requires large sample size and matched control population False-positve results in the absence

GENES AND LOCI INVOLVED IN MONI-AND POLYGENIC FORMS OF DIABETES AND HYPERTENSION

Disorder	Genes or Suceptibility Locus	Chromosomal Location	Other factors
DIABETES MELLITUS			
Monogenic forms of diabetes			
MODY 1	HNF4α (hepatocyte nuclear factor 4α)	20q12-q13.1	
MODY 1	GCK (glucokinase)	7p15-p13	
MODY 1	HNF1α (hepatocyte nuclear factor 1α)	12q24.2	
MODY 1	IPF1 (insulin promoter factor 1)	13q12.1	
MODY 5 (Renal cysts, diabetes)	INF1B* (Hepatocyte nuclear factor 1β	17cen-q21.3	
MODY 6	Nuero D1 (neurogenic differentiation factor 1)	2q32	
Loci and genes associated with susceptibility for diabetes mellitus type 2	Genes and loci identified by linkage/association studies		Diet
	CPN 10 (Calpain-10)	2q37.3	Energy expenditure
	1q,3q,8p, 12q, 20q	1q, 3q, 12,q, 20 q	Obesity
	"Candidate genes" with possible contribution		
	Peroxisome proliferator receptor gamma	3p25	
	Insulin	11p15	
	Sulfonylurea receptor	11p15.1	
	IPF1 (insulin promotor factor 1)	13q12.1	
	IRS-1 (insulin receptor substrate	2q36	
	KCNJ11 (ATP-sensitive K channel Kir6.2)	11p15.1	
	AMP1 (adiponecin)	3q27	
	PGC-1	6p21.3-p21.1	
HYPERTENSION			
Monogenic forms			
Apparent mineralocorticoid excess		11-Ketoreductase	
Glucocorticoid-remediable HTN	CYP1B1 (unequal crossover with CYP 11B2)		
Glucocorticoid-remediatble HTN	CYP11B2 (unequal crossover with CYP11B1)		
17-alpha hydroxylase deficiency	17α hydroxylase		
Liddle's syndrome	SCNN1B		
Liddle's syndrome	SCNN1G		
Pseudohypoaldosteronism type II	WNK1		
Pseudohypoaldosteronism type II	WNK4		
Early onset HTN (AD)	MR		
Early onset HTN (AD)	BBS2		
Bardet-Biedl syndrome type 2	BBS4		
Loci and genes associated with susceptibility for essential hypertension	Loci identified by linkage/association studies		Salt intake
	1p, 2p, 3p, 5p, 6q, 7q, 8q, 11q, 15q, 16q, 17q, 18q, 19p, 22q, Xp		
	"Candidate genes" with possible contribution		
	Angiotensinogen	1q42-43	
	Angiotensin converting enzyme	17q23	
	Angiotensin receptor 1	3q21-25	
	G-protein subunit 3	12p13	

METHODS USED FOR THE DETECTION OF MUTATIONS

Method	Principle	Type of Mutation Detected
COMMONLY USED TECHNIQUES		
Cytogenic analysis	Unique visual appearance of various chromosomes	Numerical or structural abnormalities in chromosomes
Fluorescent in situ hybridzation (FISH)	Hybridization to chromosomes with fluorescently labeled probes	Numerical or structural abnormalities in chromosomes
Southern blot	Hybridization with genomic probe or cDNA probe after digestion of high molecular DNA	Large deletion, insertion, rearrangement, expansions of triplet repeat, amplification
Polymerase chain reaction (PCR)	Amplification of DNA segment	Expansion of triplet repeats, variable number of tandem repeats (VNTR), gene rearrangements, translocation; prepare DNA for other mutation methods.
Reverse transcriptase PCR (RT-PCR)	Reverse transcription, amplification of DNA segment—>absence or reduction of mRNA transcription	Analyze expresed mRNA (cDNA) sequence; detect loss of expression
DNA sequencing	Direct sequencing of PCR products Sequencing of DNA segments cloned into plasmid vectors	Point mutations, small deletions, and insertions
Restriction fragment polymorphism (RFLP)	Delection of altered restriction pattern of genomic DNA (Southern blot) or PCR products	Point mutations, small deletions, and insertions
OTHER TECHNIQUES		
Single-strand conformational polymorphism (SSCP)	PCR of DNA segment; Mutations result in conformational change and altered mobility	Point mutations, small deletions, and insertions
Denaturing gradient gel electrophoresis (DGGE)	PCR of DNA segment: Mutations result in conformational change and altered mobility	Point mutations, small deletions, and insertions
RNAse cleavage	Cleavage of mismatch between mutated and wild type sequence	Point mutations, small deletions, and insertions
Oligonucleotide specific hybridization (OSH)	Hybridization of PCR products to wild type or mutated oligonucleotides immobilized on chips or slides	Point mutations, small deletions, and insertions
Microarrays	Hybridization of PCR products to wild type or mutated oligonucleotides	Point mutations, small deletions, and insertions
Protein truncation test (PTT)	Transcription/translation of cDNA isolated from tissue sample	Mutations leding to premature truncations

FREQUENCY OF CHROMOSOME ABNORMALITIES, IDENTIFIED ON THE BASIS OF ABNORMAL ULTRASOUND FINDINGS

Ultrasound Finding	Chromosomal Abnormalities (Frequency) Average, %	Range in Different Studies, %
Abnormal ultrasound	16 (nonspecific)	13-35
Omphalocele	39	26-54
Cystic hygroma	68	46-78
Congenital heart disease	30	8-40
Choroid plexus cyst	5	4-10

FREQUENCY AND DISTRIBUTION OF CHROMOSOME ABNORMALITIES IN DIFFERENT TYPES OF CLINICALLY RECOGNIZABLE PREGNANCIES

	Frequency of Abnormality			
Chromosome Abnormality	*Spontaneous Abortion*	*Stillbirth*	*Livebirth*	*Probability of to Term, %*
Trisomy, all	25.1	4.0	0.3	5
+13, 18 21	4.5	2.7	0.14	15
+16	7.5	—	—	0
Sex chromosome monosomy (45, X)	8.7	0.1	0.01	1
Triploidy	6.4	0.2	—	0
Tetraploidy	2.4	—	—	0
Structural abnormality	2.0	0.8	0.3	45
Total abnormalities	50.0	5.1	0.6	5

STUDIES OF THE PARENT AND MEIOTIC/MITOTIC STAGE OF ORIGIN OF HUMAN TRISOMIES AND SEX CHROMOSOME MONOSOMY

	Origin %				
	Paternal		*Maternal*		
	I	*II*	*I*	*II*	*Mitotic*
TRISOMY					
2	28	—	54	13	6
7	—	—	17	26	57
15	—	15	76	9	—
16	—	1	96	3	—
18	—	—	33	56	11
21	3	5	67	22	2
22	3	—	94	3	—
xxy	46	—	38	14	3
xxx	—	6	60	16	18
MONOSOMY					
X[a]	80		20		

*Results pertain to nonmosaic 45 X individuals

SOME COMONLY IDENTIFIED MICRODELETION AND MICRODUPLICATION SYNDROMES

Syndrome	Cytogenetic Location	Principal Features	Imprinting Effects
Langer-Giedion syndrome	8q24.1 (del)	Sparse hair, bulbous nose, variable mental retardation	NO
WAGR complex	11p3 (del)	Wilm's tumor, aniridia, genitourinary disorders, mental retardation	No
Beckwith-Wiedemann syndrome	11p15 (dup)	Macrosomia, macorglossia, omphalocoele	Yes, occasionally associated with "paternal uniparental disomy"
Retinoblastoma	13q14.11 (del)	Retinoblastoma due to homozygous loss of functinal RB allele	No obvious effect, although abnormal RB allele more likely to be paternal

Prader-Willi syndrome	15q11-13 (del)	Obesity, hypogonadism, mental retardation	Yes; prototypic imprinting disorder
Angelman syndrome	15q11-13 (del)	Ataxic gait	With Prader-Willi syndrome, prototypic imprinting disorder
α-Thalassemia and mental retardation	16p 13.3 (del)	α-thalassemia and mental retardation, due to deletion of distal 16p, including α-globin locus	No
Smith-Magenis syndrome	17p11.2 (del)	Brachycephaly, midface hypoplasia, mental retardation	No
Miller-Dieker syndrome	17p13 (del)	Dysmorphic facies, lissencephaly	No
Charcot-Marie-Tooth syndrome type 1A	17p11.2 (dup)	Progresive neuropathy due to microduplication	NO
DiGeorge syndrome/ velocardiofacial syndrome	22q11 (del)	Abnormalities of third and fourth branchial arches	NO

INDICATIONS FOR GENETIC COUNSELLING

Advanced maternal (>35) or paternal (>50) age
Consanguinity
Previous history of a child with birth defects or a genetic disorder
Personal or family history suggestive of a genetic disorder
High-risk ethnic groups; known carriers of genetic alterations
Documented genetic alteration in a family member
Ultrasound or prenatal testing suggesting a genetic disorder

EXAMPLES OF GENETIC TESTING AND POSSIBLE INTERVENTIONS

Genetic Disorder	Inheritance	Genes	Interventions
Herediatary nonpolyposis colon cancer	AD	MSH2, MLH1, MSH6, PMS1, PMS2	Early cancer screeing
Familial adenomatous polyposis	AD	APC	Nonsteroidal anti-inflammatory drugs Early endoscopic screening Colectomy
Familial breast and ovarian cancer	AD	BRCA1, BRCA2	Estrogen receptor antagonists Early screening by exams and mammography Consider prophylactic surgery
Familial melanoma	AD	CDKN2A Screening and biopsies	Avoid UV light
Basal cell nevus syndrome	AD	PTCH Screening and biopsies	Avoid UV light
HEMATOLOGY			
Factor V Leiden	AD	F5	Avoid thrombogenic risk factors and oral contraceptives
Hemophilia A	XL	F8C	Factor VIII replacement
Hemophilia B	XL	F9	Factor IX replacement Possible gene therapy
Glucose-6-PO4 dehydrogenease deficiency	XL	G6PD	Avoid oxidant drugs

EXAMPLES OF GENETIC TESTING AND POSSIBLE INTERVENTIONS (Contd...)

Genetic Disorder	Inheritance	Genes	Interventions
CARDIOVASCULAR			
Hypertrophic cardiomyopathy	AD	MYH7, MYBPC3, TNNT2, TPM1	Echocardiographic screening Early harmacologic intervention
Long QT syndrome	AD	KCNQ1, KCNH2, SCN5A, LQT4, KCNE1, KCNE2	Electrocardiographic screeing and electrophysiologic testing Early pharmacologic intervention Possible implantable cardioverter defibrillator
Marfan syndrome	AD	FBN1	Echocardiographic screeing Prophylactic beta blockers
GASTROINTESTINAL			
Familial Mediterranean fever	AR	MEFV	Colchicine treatment
Hemochromatosis	AR	HFE	Phlebotomy
PULMONARY			
α-1 Antitrypsin deficiency	AR	PI	Avoid smoking Avoid occupational and environmental toxins
Primary pulmonary hypertension	AD	BMPR2	Treatment with pulmonary vasodilators
RENAL			
Polycystic kidney disease	AD	PKHD1	Prevent hypertension Prevent urinary tract infections Kidney transplantation
Nephrogenic diabetes insipidus	XL,AR	AVPR2, AQP2	Fluid replacement Thiazides, amiloride
ENDOCRINE			
Neurohypophyseal diabetes insipidus	AD	AVP	Replace vasopressin
Maturity onset diabetes of the young	AD	Multiple genes	Screen and treat for diabetes
Familial hypocalciuric hypercalcemia	AD	CASR	Avoid parathyroidectomy
Kallmann syndrome	XL	KAL	Induce puberty with hormone replacement
Multiple endocrine neoplasia type 2	AD	RET	Prophylactic thyroidectomy Screen for pheochromocytoma and hyperparathyroidism
21-Hydroxylase deficiency	AR	CYP21	Glucocorticoid and mineralocorticoid treatment
NEUROLOGIC			
Malignant hyperthermia	AD	PYR1	Avoid precipitating anesthetics
Hyperkalemic periodic paralysis AD	SCN4A	Acetazolamide	
Adrenoleukodystrophy	XL	ABCD 1	Possible bone marrow transplant for severe childhood CNS form
Duchenne and Becker muscular dystrophy	XL	DMD	Glucocorticoids Possible future myoblast transfer
Familial Parkinson's disease	AD	SNCA, PARK2	Amantadine, anticholinerics, levodopa, monoamine oxidase B inhibitors
Wilson's disease	AR	ATP7B	D-Penicillamine treatment

Abbreviations : AD, autosomal dominant; AR, autosomal recessive : CNS, central nervous system: XL, X-linked

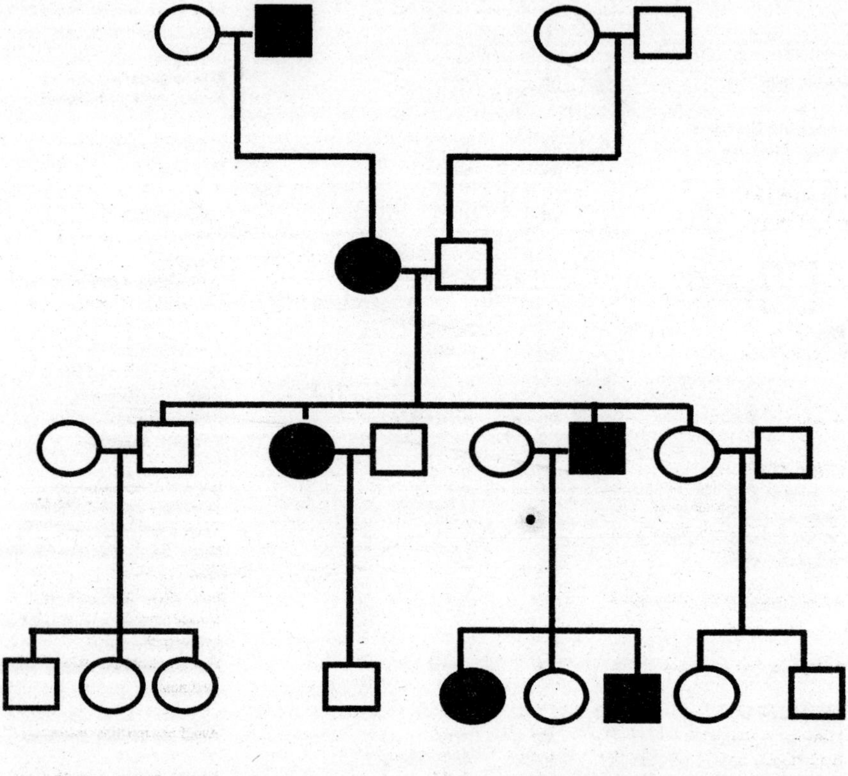

A pedigree illustrating autosomal dominant inheritance. Square symbols indicate males and circles females; open symbols indicate that the person is phenotypically unaffected, and filled symbols indicate that the phenotype is present to some extent.

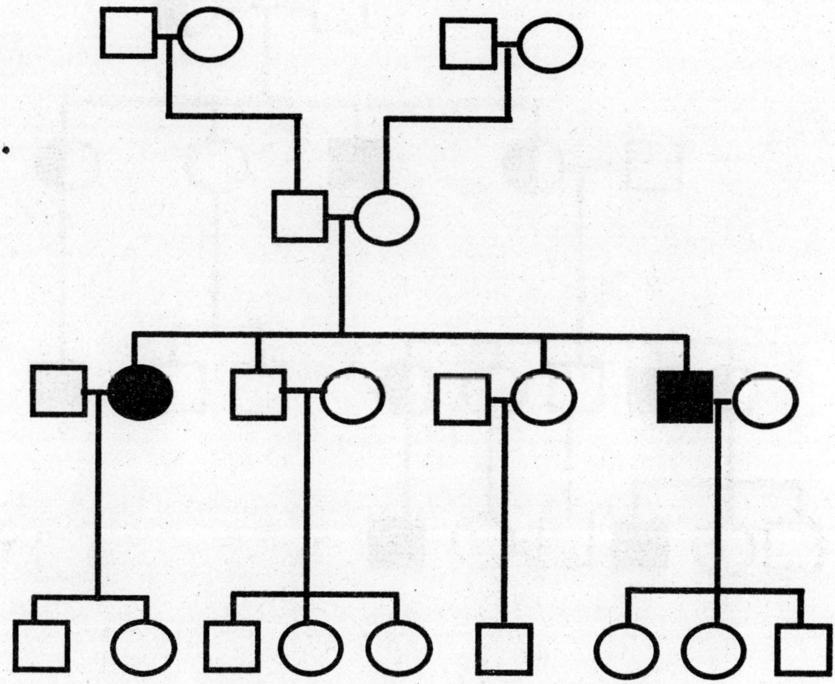

Figure : A pedigree illustrating autosomal recessive inheritance.

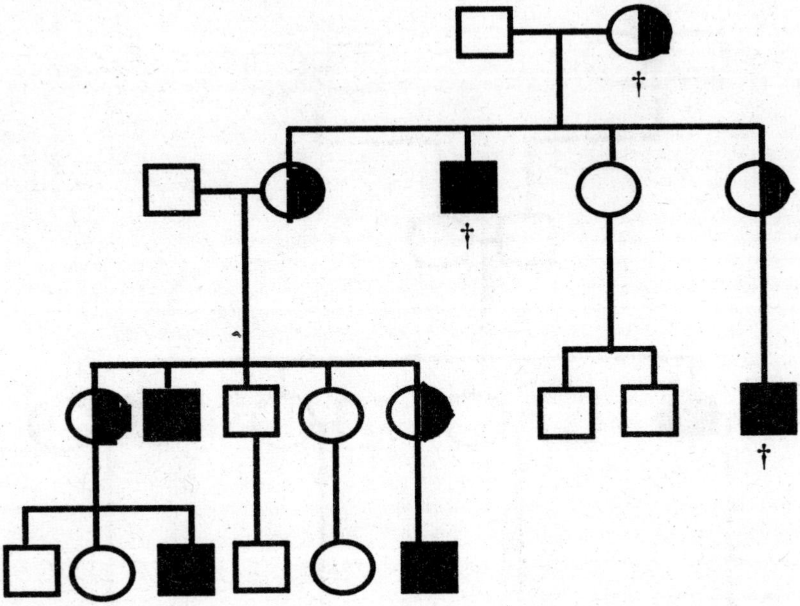

LEGEND :

 Duchenne muscular dystrophy (DMD)

 Carrier

† Deceased

X-linked recessive inheritance : Duchenne type muscular dystrophy

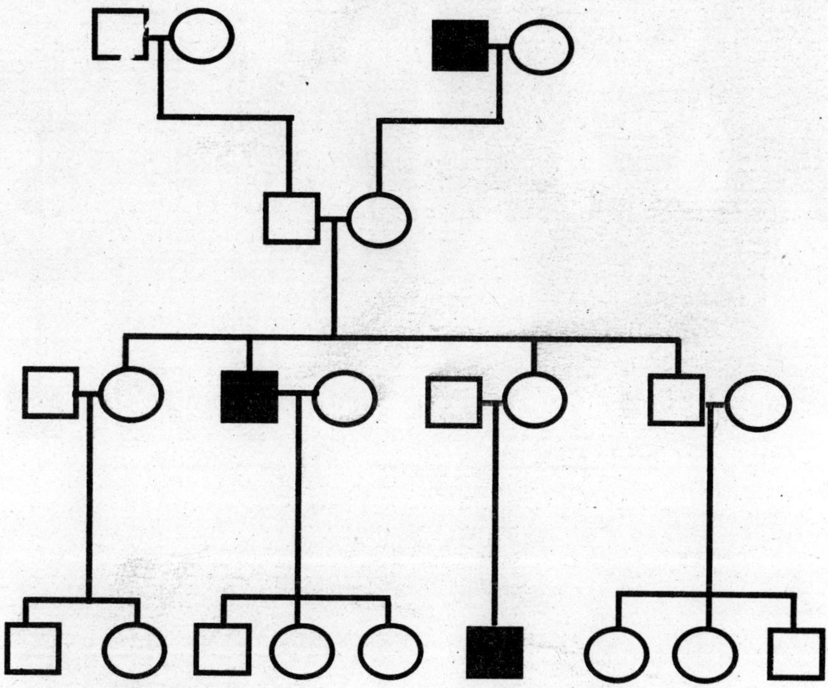

Figure : A pedigree illustrating autosomal recessive inheritance.

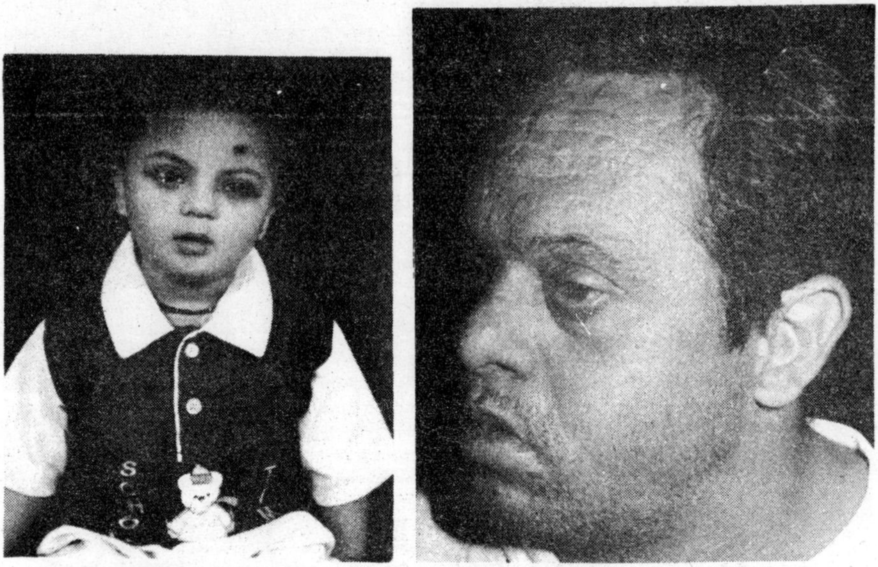

Child Adult

Fig 1. Down's syndrome

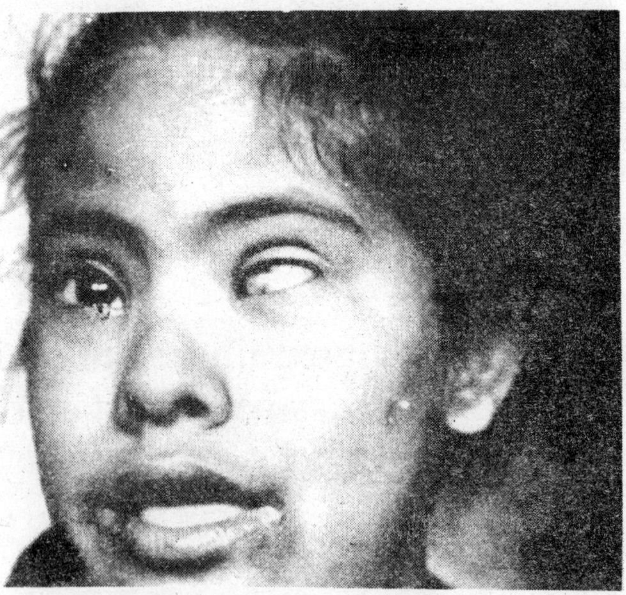

Fig 2. Congenital Rubella syndrome

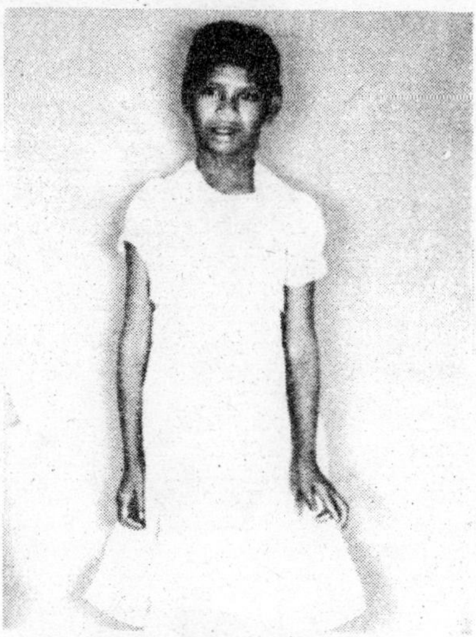

Fig 3. Short statured

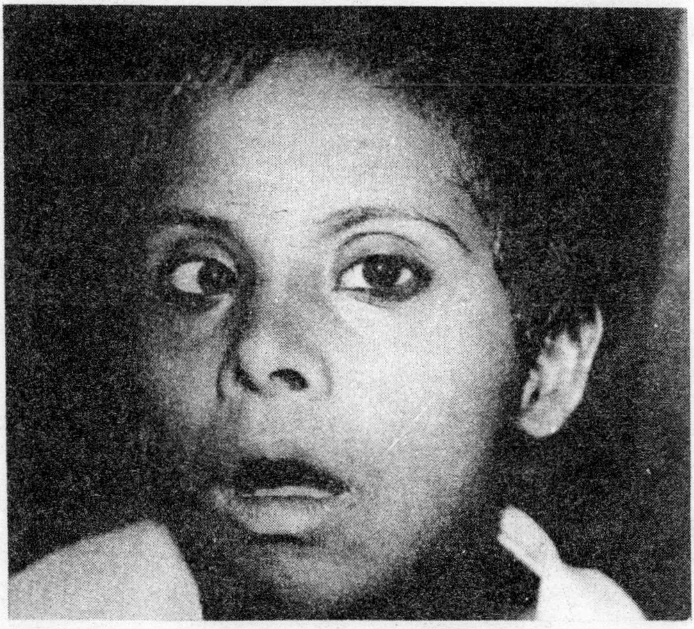

Fig 4. Mental Retardation with Microcephaly

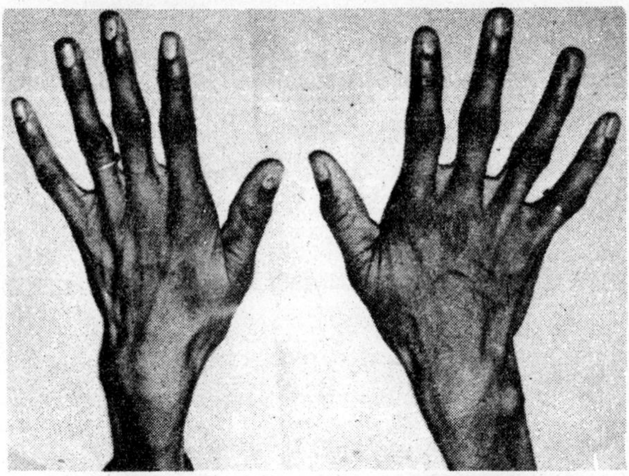

(a) Archnodactyly

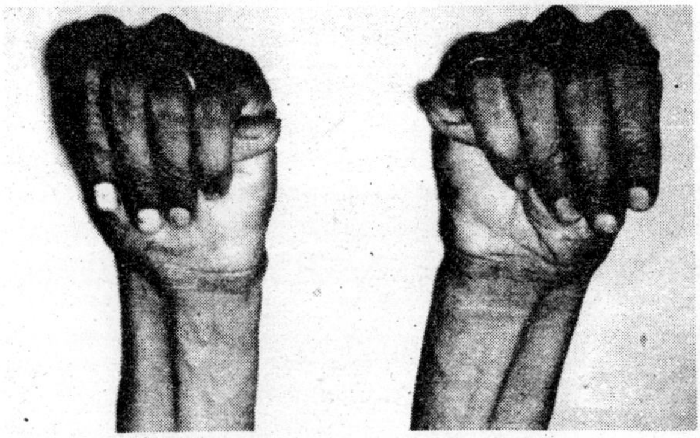

(b) Long Thumb

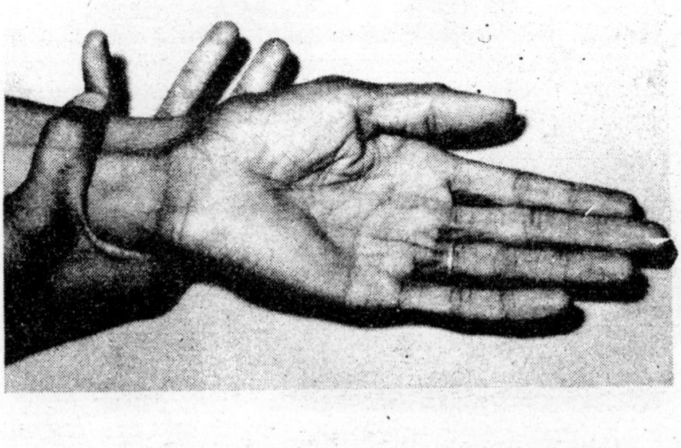

(c) Long Fingers

Fig 5. Marfan's syndrome

TERATOGENIC DRUGS

Drugs or chemical	*Teratogenic effect*
Alcohol	Cardiac, limb and facial anomalies, MR, Short stature
Lysergic acid	Skeletal anomalies (?)
Phenytoin	Facial, cardiac and limb anomalies, (±) MR, (±) Short Stature, cleft lip
Trimethadione	Facial, cardiac and visceral anomalies
Warfarin	Nasal and limb anomalies (?)
Aminopteron, methotrexete	Skeletal anomalies
Oral contraceptive	Cardiac, limb and visceral anomalies (?)
Lithium	Ebstein's anomaly
Anesthesia, general,	Respiratory depression
Anesthetics, ocal	Accidental injection into fetal scalp, fetal bradycardia acidosis, neonatal convulsions.
Analgesics; salicylates	Neonatal bleeding due to vitamin K dependent factor deficiency, reduced bilirubin binding capacity and hyperbilirubinemia.
Narcotics	Respiratory depression in the baby; withdrawal symptoms
Streptomycin	Deafness
Nitrofurantoin	Hemolysis in G-6-P-D deficient infants. Long acting sulphonamides decrease bilirubin binding capacity
Sulphonamides	
Tetracyclines	Fetal growth retardation, Staining of teeth and bones
Tolbutamide	Fetal death (?) thrombocytopenia
Sulfonylnureas	Hypoglycemia in newborn
Reserpine	Transient nasal stuffness
Quinine	Deafness, thrombocytopenia, CNS, limb anomalies
Chloroquine	Deafness (?) after prolonged use; hemolysis in susceptible individuals
Barbiturates	Withdrawal symptoms, activation of hepatic microsomal enzymes, respiratoyr depression after use in labor
Thiazides	Thrombocytopenia (?)

Iodine containing	Fetal goiter, Hypothyroidism, preparations (cough mixtures etc.)
Phenothiazines	Extrapyramidal symptoms
Androgens, synthetic progestins	Rarely masculinisation of females. Adenocarcinoma of vagina, during late adolescence
Vitamin K	Hemolytic anemia, severe neonatal jaundice
Vitamin D	Infantile hypercalcemia (?) not conculsively proven
Live virus vaccination	Vaccinia
Cigarette smoking	Low birth weight

COMMON DRUGS WHICH SHOULD BE WITHELD FROM CHILDREN WITH G-6-PD DEFICIENCY:

1. **Antimalarials**
   Primaquine
   Pamaquine
   Pentaquine
   Quinine
2. **Sulfonamides**
   Sulfonamides
   Sulfomethoxypyridazine
   Acetylsulfanilamide
   Salicylazosulfapyridazine
3. **Sulfones**
   Thiaxolsulfone
   Diaminodiphenylsulfone (DDS)
4. **Analgesics and antipyretics**
   Antipyrine
   Amidopyrine
   Aminosalicylic acid
5. **Antibiotics**
   Streptomycin
6. **Antituberculous drugs**
   Isoniazid
   Para-aminosalicylic acid

7. **Chemotherapeutic agents**
   Nitrofurantion
   Furazolidine
   Nitrofurazone
   Phenylhydrazine
   Phenytoin sodium
8. **Antidiabetic agents**
   Tolbutamide
   Chlorpropamide
9. **Miscellaneous**
   Water soluble vitamin analogues
   Naphtalene
   Probenecid
   Arsenic compounds
   Fava beans

DRUGS WHICH CAN BE USED WITH CAUTION G-6-PD INDIVIDUALS. (DRUGS SHOULD PREFERABLY BE USED IN LOWER DOSAGES. THESE DRUGS CAUSE HEMOLYSIS LESS FREQUENTLY)

---

1. **Antimalarials**
   Chloroquine
   Mepacrine
2. **Sulfonamides**
   Sulfadiazine
   Sulfafurazole
3. **Analgesics and antipyretics**
   Acetylsalicylic acid
   Phenacetin
4. **Antibiotics**
   Chloramphenicol
5. **Others**
   Ascorbic acid (high doses)
   Methylene blue
   Dimercaprol

DRUGS WHICH ARE EXCREATED IN BREAST MILK AND PRODUCE ADVERSE EFFECTGS ON NURSING INFACTS

1. **Anticonvulsants and desatives**
   Diazepam
   Carbamazepine
   Chlorpromazine
   Lithium Carbonate
   Ethanol
2. **Anticoagulants**
   Phenindione
   Ethylbiscoumarate
3. **Hormones and related drugs**
   Iodides
   Thyroxine
   Thiouracil
   Spironolactone
   Dihydrotachysterol
   Oral contraceptive(?)
   Prednisone and prednisolone (?)
4. **Radioactive drugs**
   It is advisable to stop breast for at least 10-14 days after a radio-isotope study in the mother.
5. **Antimetabolites**
6. **Antibiotics**
   Tetracycline
   Chloramphenicol
7. **Miscellaneous**
   Metronidazole
   Ergot alkaloids
   Bromides
   Phenophthalein
   Reserpine

ORIGINAL SOLVED MCQ's IN DM CLINICAL GENETICS

1. **Genetic information of nuclear DNA is transmitted to the site of protein synthesis by :**
   A. Polysomes B. tRNA
   C. rRNA D. mRNA
2. **Jacob and Monod postulated that enzymes inducers exert their effect by increacting with :**
   A. Operator gene B. Repressor protein
   C. Structural gene D. Regularatory metabolite
   E. Aminoacyl tRNA
3. **At certain pH amino acid behaves neither as an acid nor as a base and does not migrate to anode or chatode is called —— :**
   A. Nitrogenous equillibrium
   B. Isoelectric point
   C. Zwitterion
   D. None of the above
4. **Base stacking of DNA is by :**
   A. Linear dichromicity B. Hypochromicity
   C. Hyperchromicity D. Electrophoresis
5. **All the following apply to mutations except one :**
   A. Changes in base sequnece of DNA
   B. May lead to synthesis of defective DNA polymerase
   C. Are caused by chemical mutagens only
   D. May result of decreasd synthesis of enxyme proteinase
6. **'Chargaff rule states that :**
   A. A + G = T + C B. A/T = G/C
   C. A = U = T = G = C D. A + T = G + C
7. **Degeneracy of the genetic code denotes the existence of :**
   A. Multiple codons for a single amino acid
   B. Codons consisting of only two bases
   C. Base triplets that do not code for any amino acid
   D. Different codons for the same amino acid but contain unusual bases

Ans. 1. D 2. B 3. B 4. C 5. C 6. B 7. A

8. **The term modified base refers to :**
   A. Purine or pyrimidine attached to deoxyribose
   B. A purine or pyrimidine that has been altered
   C. A nitrogen containing ring other than a pruien or pyrimidine that is part of accucleotide
   D. A purine or pyrimidine attached to a sugar by o-glycoside linkage
9. **In DNA, 2 strands are held by :**
   A. Covalent bonds B. Coordinate bonds
   C. Metalic bonds D. Hydrogen bonds
10. **In reverse transcription, mRNA uses template :**
    A. Single stranded DNA B. Double stranded DNA
    C. Ribosomes D. rRNA
11. **DNA exist in vivo mainly as a :**
    A. Left handed b-helix B. Right handed a-helix
    C. Right handed b-helix D. Left handed a-helix
12. **Banding is :**
    A. Method of detecting single gene deletion
    B. Fluorescene filters are used
    C. Y chromosome in seen in interphase
    D. Trypsin and Giemsa are used
13. **Maximum no. of H bonds are found between which base pairs ?**
    A. A-T B. G-C
    C. A-G D. C-T
14. **Northern blot test is used for :**
    A. DNA analysis B. RNA analysis
    C. Analysis of proteins D. Enzyme analysis
15. **Replacement of a codon coding for an aminoacid by another codon coding for another aminoacid results in :**
    A. Missense mutation B. Mutagen
    C. Somatic mutation D. Miscoding
16. **The intermediate that conveys information from the nucleus to the cytoplasm in eukaryotes is :**
    A. tRNA B. mRNA
    C. rRNA D. RNA polymerase
17. **Of prime importance in the structure of flavoproteins is :**
    A. Vit B6 B. VIt B2
    C. Vit B1 D. Vit A
18. **Independent DNA replication occurs in all except :**
    A. Bacteria B. Mitochondria
    C. Nuclei D. Viruses

Ans.	8. B	9. D	10. A	11. C	12. A	13. B
	14. B	15. A	16. D	17. B	18. D	

19. After translation, product formed is :

A. mRNA B. t-TNA
C. r-RNA D. Protein

20. Which is the purine nuceloside ?

A. Adenosine B. Cytidine
C. Thymidine D. Uracil

21. Which is the pyrimidine nucleoside ?

A. Guanine 5 phosphate B. Adenosine
C. Deoxythymidine D. Cytosine

22. Which of the following is not a constitutent of gangliosidic molecules :

A. Glycerol B. Sialic acid
C. Lecithins D. Long-chain fatty acid

23. To obtain double stranded cDNA from mRNA the enzyme involved is :

A. DNA polymerase B. Reverse transcriptase
C. Ligase D. Polymerase II

24. Sources of the nucleotide portion of NAD include :

A. N-methyl nicotinamide B.The vitamin riboflavin
C. PRPP D. Tryptophan

25. Which of the following is a precursor fo protoporphyrin?

A. Leucine B. Alanine
C. Proline D. Histidine
E. Glycine

26. If the percentage of adenine in a double stranded DNA molecule is 20%, the percentage of guanine is :

A. 0% B. 10%
C. 20% D. 30%

27. Which of the following into the polypeptide incorporated directly into the polypeptide chain during the translation of mRNA :

A. Asparagine B. Homoserine
C. 4-hydroxyproline D. Phosphoserine

28. Which of the following amino acid is nto specific for sugar attachment in glycoproproteins :

A. Proline B. Serine
C. Asparagine D. Hydroxy proline

29. All of the following enzymes are involved in the excision repair of DNA except :

A. DNA ligase B. DNA glycocyclase
C. Exonuclease D. DNA β-polymerase

Ans.	**19. B**	**20. A**	**21. C**	**22. A**	**23. B**	**24. D**
	25. E	**26. D**	**27. A**	**28 C**	**29. C**	

Questions 90 and 91

A. Replication
B. Transcription
C. Translation
D. Postranslational modification
E. Glycosylation

30. **DNA-dependent RNA synthesis**
31. **Ribosokal protein synthesis**

Questions 92 to 95

A. DNA
B. Ribosomal RNA
C. Transfer RNA
D. Messenger RNA
E. 5S RNA

32. **CCA occurs at the 3' ednd :**
33. **Introns are removed in spliting reaction following polydenylation reaction :**
34. **Capped by 7-methylgunosine :**
35. **Produced in the nucleus :**
36. **Amino acid sequence of a polypeptide is fundamentally determined by :**
    A. Base sequence of tRNA
    B. Base sequence of mRNA
    C. Base sequence of DNA
    D. Double stranded RNA
37. **In mammalian cells protein sequence takes place chiefly at the :**
    A. Smooth endoplasmic reticulum
    B. Rough endoplasmic reticulum
    C. Nucleus
    D. Lysosomes
38. **Xeroderma pigmentosum, a rate skin disease is due to an autosomal recessive trait which causes a defi-ciency of :**
    A. DNA polymerase
    B. DNA-dependent RNA polymerase
    C. DNA ligase
    D. A specific DNA endonuclease
39. **The degradation of RNA by pancreatic ribonuclease produces :**
    A. Nuceloside 2' phosphates
    B. Nucleoside 3' phosphates
    C. Nucleoside 5' phosphates
    D. Nucleotides

Ans.	30. B	31. C	32. C	33. D	34. D	35. B
	36. C	37. B	38. D	39. B		

40. The Watson Crick model of DNA strands running in opposite directions :

A. Double DNA strands running in opposite directions
B. A triple-stranded structure
C. Pair bonding between bases A and G
D. Covalent bonding between bases

41. The first step in the utilization of aminoacids for protein sysnthesis requres the :

A. Arginyl-RNA synthetase
B. Amino-acyl soluble RNA synthetase
C. Amino acid activating enzyme
D. Chain initiating enzyme

42. The smallest unit of DNA capable of regulating the synthesis of a polypeptide is the :

A. Operon B. Cistron
C. Recon D. Muton

43. The percentage of a bacterial chromosome usually involved in transformation is :

A. 1 percent B. 10 percent
C. 25 perc

44. A codon consists of :

A. 2 complementary base pairs
B. 3 complementary base pairs
C. 4 complementary base paris
D. 4 individual nucleotides

45. Acitinomycin D interfers with enzyme induction by combining with :

A. t-RNA
B. r-RNA
C. DNA
D. Negative feedback inhibition system

46. JacoB and Monod postulated that enzyme inducers exert their effect by interacting with :

A. Strucutrla gene B. Operator gene
C. Repressor gene D. Aminoacyl RNA

47. Nucleotide is :

A. Sugar + Phosphate B. Sugar + Base
C. Base + Phosphate D. Base + Sugar + Phosphate

48. Which of the following contains the anticodon :

A. DNA B. Ribosomal RNA
C. Messenger RNA D. Transfer RNA

Ans.	40. A	41. C	42. B	43. A	44. B	45. C
	46. B	47. D	48. D			

49. Which of the following is the initiating amino acid for protein synthesis :

A. Alanine
B. Methionine
C. Serine
D. Lysine
E. Cysteine

50. The initating codon for protein synthesis is :

A. AUG
B. UAA
C. UUU
D. UAG

51. 5' GCT 3' DNA when converted into RNA presents as :

A. 5' CGA 3'
B. 5' AGC 3'
C. 5' CGU 3'
D. 5' UGC 3'

52. Both the carbon and the nitrogen atoms of which of the following are directly incorporated into purines during their biosynghesis :

A. Glutamine
B. Aspartate
C. Glycine
D. Asparagine

53. Coproporyphyrin III is : (Hb) :

A. Normal hemoglolin breakdown product
B. Normal Hb precursor
C. Excreted in lead poisoning
D. Excreted in hepatic porphyria

54. Which of the following is a precursor of photoporphyrin :

A. Alanine
B. Leucine
C. Histidine
D. Glycine

55. Which of the following is a substrate for ribonucleo-tide reductase in the production of deoxyribonucleo-tides in humans?

A. ATP
B. AMP
C. TDP
D. GTP

56. Whic of the following sequences of DNA and its complement constitutes a palindrome ?

A. AAAA
B. AATT
C. ATTA
D. AAAT

57. In phospholipids of cephalin type, choline is replaced by :

A. Serine
B. Inositol
C. Betain
D. Ethanolamine serine and inositol

58. The type of RNA that characteristically contains methylated purines and pyrimidines is :

A. mRNA
B. t-RNa
C. r-RNA
D. All of the above

Ans.	49. B	50. A	51. A	52. C	53. C	54. D
	55. D	56. B	57. D	58. B		

58. The attachmeni site of DNA-Dependent RNA polymerse to a gene is the :

A. Operator B. Promoter
C. Structural gene D. Regulatory gene

60. In sickle cell anaemia, the defect can be explained as having arisen from :

A. A base insertion in DNA
B. A base deletion in DNA
C. A base substitution in DNA
D. None of the above

61. Which of the following nucelic acid bases is found in mRNA but not in DNA :

A. Adenine B. Cystosine
C. Guanine D. Uracil

62. Uric acid synthesis in mammals takes place in :

A. Bone marrow B. Muscle
C. Liver D. Liver and kidney

63. Conversion of a UMP to TMP requires :

A. ATP B. Tetrahydrofolic acid
C. FMN D. Pyridoxal phosphate

64. The four nitrogen atoms of purines are derived from :

A. Aspartate, glutamine and glycine
B. Glycine and aspartate
C. Urea and ammonia
D. Glycine, glutamate and ammonia

65. Complete acid hydrolysis of nucelic acids will not yelds :

A. Ribose B. Guanine
C. Phosphate D. Adenosine

66. AdenyDic acid is synthesized by reactions involving :

A. Inosinic acid + NAD ++ glutamine
B. Inosinic acid + GTP + aspartate
C. Inosinic acid + NH3
D. Ribose-1-PO4+ hypoxanthine

67. A key substance in pyridine biosynthesis is :

A. ATP B. Thiouracil
C. Carbamoyl phosphate D. Ribose-5-PO4
E. NADP+

68. Nucleoproteins are conjugated proteins containing nucleic acid and :

A. Albuminoid proteins B. Scleroproteins
C. Glycoproteins D. Protamines or histones

Ans.	59. B	60. C	61. D	62. C	63. B	64. A
	65. D	66. B	67. C	68. D		

69. Inosinic acid is biological precursor of :
A. Uracil and thymine
B. Purines and pyridmidines
C. Adenylic acid and guanylic acid
D. Orotic acid and uridylic acid

70. The two polynucleotide chains of DNA double helix :
A. Are connected by disulfide bonds
B. Are held together by phosphate diester bonds
C. Cannot be separated
D. Differ in chemical composition

71. Two hydrogen bonds are seen between :
A. A & T
B. A & C
C. U & C
D. G & C

72. Which term describes protiens produced by a muta-tion of an operon causing uncon-trolled operation of genes distal to it :
A. Deleted
B. Constitutive
C. Repressed
D. Augmented
E. Derepressed

73. Most active site of protein synthesis is the :
A. Cell sap
B. Mitochndrion
C. Ribosome
D. Nucleus

74. The committed step in pyrimidine biosynthesis :
A. Catalyzed by orotate decarboxylase
B. Required ATP
C. In formation of N-carbamolaspartic acid
D. Results in formation of dihydroorotic acid

75. Pyrimidines besides occuring in nucleic acids, are found in :
A. Flavine meononucleotide
B. Thiamine
C. Uric acid
D. Adenine

76. RNA does not contain :
A. Uracil
B. Phosphate
C. Ribose
D. Dydroxymethylcytosine

77. A phosphoribosyl transferase catalyses the following reaction :
A. Purine + Ribose -1-PO4—>Nucleoside
B. Purine + ATP → Nucleotide
C. Purine + Phosphoribosyl pyrophosphate→Nucleotide
D. None of the above

78. DNA may be easily distinguishable from RNA by :
A. Measurement of their ultraviolet spectra
B. Extraction of DNA by hot trichloro-acetic acid
C. Colour reaction for the specific sugar
D. Estimation of rate of trypsin digestion

Ans.	69. C	70. D	71. A	72. B	73. C	74. C
	75. B	76. D	77. C	78. C		

79. **5-phosphoribosyl-1-pyrophosphate is an inter-mediate in the synthesis of :**
A. NAD+ B. Purines
C. Purine nucleotides D. Pyrimidine nucelotides
E. All of the above

80. **Melanin pigment is increased by all except :**
A. Arachidonic acid B. Prostaglandins
C. Heavy metals D. U-V rays

81. **Which of the following is called the second messenger :**
A. cAMP B. cGMP
C. NADP D. a + b

82. **Which colour indicates positive xanthoproteic reaction :**
A. Yellow B. Blue
C. Red D. Puple

83. **All of the following carriers are components of the mitochondrial electron transport chain except :**
A. NAD
B. NADP
C. Flavinmononucleotide
D. Flavin adenine dinucleotide

84. **Which vitamin is the most indispensable during mitosis :**
A. Folic acid B. Pantothenic acid
C. Ascorbic acid D. Aspartic acid

85. **t-RNA, true is :**
A. Inverted T-appearence
B. Each specific for one RNA
C. No Intra basal pairing
D. Clover leaf pattern

86. **What results due to incomplete oxidation of phenylpyruvic acid :**
A. Phenylketonuria B. Albinism
C. Tyroinosis D. Alkaptonuria

87. **Which of the following is not present in RNA :**
A. Adenine B. Thymine
C. Uracil D. Guanine

88. **Which is not possible :**
A. G-C B. A-T
C. A-U D. A-G

89. **Chain terminator codons are all except :**
A. AUG B. UGA
C. UAG D. UAA

Ans.	79. E	80. C	81. D	82. A	83. B	84. A
	85. D	86. A	87. B	88. D	89. A	

90. Gene transmitted but not translated is :

A. Histone B. Keratin
C. t-RNA D. Glycosyl

91. In RNA gene during processing undergoes all except :

A. Nuclease cleavage B. Nucleoside modifications
C. Terminate additions D. Chemical hydrolysis

92. DNA polymerase is used in the following :

A. Magnifies small fragment of DNA
B. Splenic cell culture
C. Mano cell culture
D. All of the above

93. Protein synthesis - N. of AA is arranged by :

A. t-RNA restriction B. DNA restriction
C. mRNA restriction D. rTNA restriction

94. Messenger RNA attaches to which of the following for regulating protein synthesis :

A. Operator codon B. Terminator codon
C. Soluble RNA D. DNA

95. Which of the following radiolabelled bases identify well the DNA and not the RNA :

A. Adenine B. Thymine
C. Porphyrin D. Uracil

96. RNA split is at :

A. Nucleoside-5-phosphate
B. Nucleoside 1,5 diphosphate
C. Nucleoside triphosphate
D. Any of the above

97. Cytosine is analogue to :

A. Thymine B. Uracil
C. Adenine D. Guanine

98. All are true about ribosomal RNA except :

A. Forms major part of RNA
B. Does protein synthesis
C. In Eukaryotes two types are seen - 60 S & 40 S
D. In man two types are seen 70 S & 50 S

99. All are true about DNA except :

A. Its stands are bonded by disulfide bonds
B. Adenine corresponds to thymine
C. Guanine corresponds to cytosine
D. Nucleotide consists of a purine base, deoxyribose sugar & phosphoric acid

Ans.	90. A	91. D	92. C	93. B	94. A	95. B
	96. A	97. B	98. D	99. A		

100. Enzyme utilized n virus replication is :
A. DNA dependent RNA polymerase
B. RNA dependent DNA polymerase
C. Restrictive endonuclease
D. DNA dependent DNA polymerase

101. RNA synthesis is determined by radio activity using :
A. C 14 uridine B. H 3 thymine
C. N 15 uridine D. P 32 Phosphate

102. Unwinding of DNA is done by :
A. DNAse I B. Topoisomerase I
C. Ligase D. Restriction endonuclease

103. `Leucine zipper' motif is a mediator for :
A. Membrane attack complexes
B. Receptor Ligand Protein
C. Binding of regulatory proteins of DNA
D. B-cell epitopes

104. Proof reading of m-RNA is done by :
A. Peptidyl transferase B. Aminoacyl transferase
C. Formulase D. RNA polymerase type I

105. UV rays causes :
A. Deletion of pyramidines
B. Substitution of purines for pyramidine
C. Cross linking of purine with pyrimidine
D. Dimensation of pyramidine

106. Chromomeres are rich in :
A. RNA B. DNA
C. Protein D. All

107. Following are true about DNA - B except :
A. It contain 10 base pair per turn
B. Both chains are parallels to each other
C. Between two base pairs there is hydrogen bond
D. A+T=G+C

108. The following base sequence and its complementary sequence are palindromic :
A. AAAA B. AATT
C. AAGG D. GTGT

109. Gene that is involved in transcription but excluded before translation are :
A. Extrons B. Introns
C. Preinitiation complex D. Initiator sequence

Ans.	100. B	101. A	102. B	103. C	104. B	105. D
	106. D	107. B	108. B	109. B		

110. In Gene cloning, largest segment is :

A. Plasmid B. Cosmid
C. Bacteriophage D. Beta globulin

111. Triplex helix is seen in :

A. Collegen B. DNA
C. Pectin D. Cystine

112. Okazaki fragments are short pieces of DNA replicated :

A. Continuously in the 5'-3' direction
B. Discontinuously in the 3'-5' direction
C. Continuously in the 3'-5' direction
D. Discontinuously in the 5'-3' direction

113. Degeneracy of the genetic code denotes the existance of :

A. Condons consisting of only two bases
B. Condons that include one or more of the unusual bases
C. Multiple condons for a single amino acid
D. Base triplets coding for different amono acids

114. Consider the following statements :
Chargaffs observation on nitrogen base contents of DNA of all sepcies is that there are equal numbers of:

1. Adenine and guanine 2. Adenine and thymine
3. Guanine and cytosine 4. Guanine and thymine

Of these statements

A. 1 and 2 are correct B. 2 and 3 are correct
C. 3 and 4 are correct D. 1 and 4 are correct

115. Post-translational hydroxylation of uracil forms thymine in :

A. Messenger RNA B. Transfer RNA
C. Ribosomal RNA D. Heteronuclear RNA

116. Which one of the following is not a termination codon ?

A. UCU B. UAA
C. UGA D. UAG

117. In post-transcriptional processing of m-RNA, "splicing" refers to :

A. Joining exons after the removal of introns
B. Addition of exons to m-RNA
C. Addition of introns to m-RNA
D. Removal of exons and joining introns

118. The melting temperature (Tm) of DNA is related to the :

A. Length of the two strands of DNA
B. Type of the double helix present in DNA
C. Base composition of DNA
D. Diameter of the double helix of DNA

Ans.	110. B	111. A	112. A	113. C	114. B	115. B
	116. A	117. A	118. C			

119. Consider the following statements :
DNA fingerprint is valuable in
1. Determination of blood group
2. Investigation of crime
3. Investigation of autoimmune
4. Determination of paternity

Of these statements :
A. 1 and 3 are correct B. 3 and 4 are correct
C. 2 and 4 are correct D. 1and 2 are correct

120. Which one of the following is the function of "small nuclear ribonucleoprotein particles (SnRNP) ?
A. Initiation of protein synthesis
B. Activation of amino acids
C. Processing of RNA
D. Replication of DNA

121. Function of endonuclease :
A. Cut DNA at specific DNA sequences
B. To point out the coding regions
C. Enhancers
D. To find out antibiotic resistance

122. Genetic information originates from :
A. Cistrons of DNA
B. Anticodons of tRNA
C. Histones of nucleoproteins
D. Codons of mRNA

123. What is the function of the acceptor arm of tRNA moleucles ?
A. It binds with specific amino acids to form aminoacyl tRNA
B. It helps in the recognition of the codon of mRNA
C. It helps in the transfer of mRNA from the neucleus to the cytoplasm
D. It binds with the initiation factors to form the initiation complex during protein synthesis

124. The codons code for the same amino acid in all organisms. Therefore they are :
A. Non overlapping B. Degenerate
C. Universal D. Unambiguous

125. Which one of the following sub-units of a ribosome binds to the mRNA to initiate protein synthesis ?
A. 60 S B. 60 S-GTP complex
C. 40S D. 40 S-ATP complex

Ans.	119. C	120. C	121. A	122. A	123. A	124. C
	125. A					

126. Pentose sugars are physiologically important because ribose and deoxyribase sugars are part of nucelic acids. Name the vitamins which has a ribose sugar in its structure :

A. Folic acid B. Riboflavin
C. Niacin D. Cyanocobalamine

127. α helix and b pleated arrangement in a protein is seen in ——— structure :

A. Primary B. Secondary
C. Tertiary D. Quatermery

128. On complete hydrolysis of DNA we will get all the following except :

A. Deoxy pentose sugar B. Phosphoric acid
C. Adenosine D. Purine bases

129. Which of the following RNA has abnormal purine bases :

A. tRNA B. mRNA
C. rRNA D. 16S RNA

130. True statement about synthesis of eukaryotic RNA is :

A. Consist of 2 helical strands
B. Synthesized from DNA by RNA polymerase
C. Ribosomal RNA is synthesized and forms ribosome in cytoplasm
D. Proteins are synthesized in nucleus from mRNA and released into cytoplasm

131. True statement about nuclear DNA is :

A. Purine and pyrimidine content is equal
B. Replication of DNA occurs by enzyme DNA polymerase
C. Consists of two helical strands bound by hydrogen bonds
D. All of the above

132. Total number of genes in human being is :

A. 30000 B. 50000
C. 100000 D. 3000000

133. Largest group of Mendalian disorders is :

A. AD B. AR
C. XR D. XD

134. All these diseases are due to triplet repeat sequences except :

A. Alzheimers B. Huntington's chorea
C. Fragile X D. Myotonic dystrophy

135. Which method is used for reading large chr 50-100 base pairs :

A. RFLP B. Chromosome walking
C. PCR D. None

Ans.	**126. D**	**127. B**	**128. C**	**129. A**	**130. B**	**131. D**
	132. A	**133. A**	**134. A**	**135. A**		

136. An alpha helix of a protein is most likely to be disrupted if a missense mutation introduces the following amino acid within the alpha helical structure :

A. Alanine B. Aspartic acid
C. Tyrosine D. Glycine

137. At the physiological pH, the DNA molecules are :

A. Positively charged B. Negatively charged
C. Neutral D. Amphipathic

138. The protein rich in basic aminoacids, which functions in the packaging of DNA in chromosomes is :

A. Histone
B. Collagen
C. Hyaluronic acid binding protein
D. Fibrinogen

139. Which of the following is not a post transcriptional modification of RNA :

A. Splicing B. 5' capping
C. 3' polyadenylation D. Glycosylation

140. Restriction fragment length polymorphism is used for :

A. Analysis of chromosome structure
B. DNA estimation
C. Synthesis of nucleic acid
D. Detecting proteins in a cell

141. Replication and transcription are similar processes in mechanistic terms because both :

A Use RNA primers for initiation.
B Use decoxybonucleotides as precursors.
C Are semi conserved events
D Involve phosphodiester bond formation with elongation occurring in the 5' - 3' direction.

142. Shine - Dalgarno sequence in bacterial mRNA is near?

A. AUG codon B. UAA codon
C. UAG codon D. UGA codon

143. An enzyme that makes a double stranded DNA copy from a single stranded RNA template molecule is known as?

A. DNA polymerase B. RNA polymerase
C. Reverse transcriptase D. Phosphokinase

144. A segment of an eucaryotic gene that is not represented in the mature mRNA, is known as?

A. Intron B. Exon
C. Plasmid D. TATA box

Ans.	136. B	137. B	138. A	139. D	140. A	141. B
	142. A	143. C	144. A			

145. RNA polymerase does not require?
A. Template (dsDNA)
B. Activated precursors (ATP, CTP, UTP, CTP)
C. Divalent metal ions (Mn^{2+}, Mg^{2+})
D. Primer

146. The following are tumor markers except :
A. Albumin B. Thyroglobulin
C. AFP D. CEA

147. Genetically determined tumours inlclude the following except :
A. Polyposis cell B. Retinoblastoma
C. Multiple neurofibroma D. Neuroblastoma

148. Aneuploidy is due to :
A. Non-dysjunction at meiosis
B. Mosaicism
C. Deletion
D. Translocation

149. The gene coding for HLA antigen is present on :
A. 6 p B. 6 q
C. 16 p D. 16 q

150. Mapping of chromosome according to form and number is as:
A. Genotyping B. Chromosome bonding
C. Phenotyping D. Karyotyping

151. All are tumour suppressor genes except:
A. Mad mạx gene B. Retinoblastoma gene
C. P53 gene D. N - mic gene

152. Sera used for HLA typing by cytotoxicity assay are obtained from all of the following sources, except :
A. Multiparous women
B. Rabbits immunized with human lymphocytes
C. Patients who have received and rejected transplanted grafts
D. Volunteers who have been HLA sensitized

153. Deletion of short arm of chromosome 11 is seen in :
A. Osteosarcoma B. Meningioma
C. Wilms tumor D. Colon Ca

154. All are true about HLA complex except :
A. Class I antigen are expressed in all nucleated cells and platelets.
B. Class II inducts helper T-cells
C. Class I is homodiamer whereas Class II is heterodiamer
D. Class I inducts cytotoxic T-cells

Ans.	145. D	146. A	147. D	148. A	149. A	150. D
	151. A	152. B	153. C	154. C		

155. The tumor suppressor gene present in head and neck tumors is :

A. P43 B. P53
C. P63 D. P73

156. Not a tumor marker :

A. Tartarate resistant alkaline phosphatase
B. CEA
C. AFP
D. Alpha-1 antitrypsin

157. The gene that regulates normal morphogenesis during development is :

A. FMR-1 gene B. Homoeobox gene
C. P-16 D. PTEN

158. Which of the following procedures are used as routine technique for karyotyping using light microscopy ?

A. C-banding B. G-banding
C. Q-banding D. BrdV-staining

159. A 60- years man presented with fatigue weight loss and heaviness in left hypochodrium for 6 months. The hemogram showed Hb 10 gm/dL, TLC 5 laks/mm3, platelet count 4 laks/mm3 , DLC; neutrophil 55%, lymphocytes 4% montocytes 2 % basophiles 6% meta-myelocytes 10% myeloytes 18%, promyelocytes 2% and blasts 3%. The most likely cytogenetic abnormality in this case is :

A. t (8; 21). B. t (9; 22).
C. t (15; 17). D. trisomy 21.

160. Which of the following is the feature of Y chromosome?

A. Acrocentric B. Telocentric
C. Submetacentric D. Metacentric

161. Males who are sexually underdeveloped with rudimentary testes and prostate glands, sparse pubic and facial hair, long arms and legs and large hands and feet are likely to have the chromosome complement of?

A. 46, XYY B. 46, XY
C. 46, XXY D. 46, X

162. Kinky-hair disease is a disorder where an affected child has peculiar white stubby hair, does not grow, brain degeneration is seen and dies by age of two years. Mrs. A is hesitant about having children because her two sisters had sons who had died from kinky hair disease. Her mother's brother also died of the same condition. Which of the following is the possible mode of inheritance in her family?

A. X-linked recessive B. X-linked dominant
C. Autosomal recessive D. Autosomal dominant

Ans.	155. B	156. D	157. B	158. B	159. B	160. A
	161. C	162. A				

163. In which of the following conditions the level of creatinine kinase-I increases?

A. Myocardial Ischemia B. Brain Ischemia
C. Kidney damage D. Electrical cardioversion

164. To which of the following events the good outcome in Neuroblastoma is associated with ?

A. Diploidy B. N-myc amplification
C. Chromosome 1 p deletion D. Trk A expression

165. Which of the following is an autosomal dominant metabolic disorder?

A. Cystic fibrosis
B. Phenylketonuria
C. a-1-antitrypsin deficiency
D. Familial hypercholesterolemia

166. Which of the following is an antiapoptotic gene ?

A. C-myc B. P53
C. bcl-2 D. bax

167. Which of the following is the most common cytogenetic abnormality in adult Myelodysplastic syndrome (MDS)?

A. Trisomy 8 B. 20 q-
C. 5q D. Monosomy 7

168. A 40 year old man presented with painless haematuria. Bimanual examination revealed a ballotable mass over the right flank. Subsequently right nephrectomy was done and the mass was seen to be composed of cells with clear cytoplasm. Areas of haemorrhage and necrosis were frequent. Cytogenetic analysis of this mass is likely to reveal the abnormality of ?

A. Chromosome 1 B. Chromosome 3
C. Chromosome 11 D. Chromosme 17

169. The commonest site of oral cancer among Indian population is ?

A. Tongue B. Floor of mouth
C. Alveobuccal complex D. Lip

170. An exmple of a tumour suppressor gene is :

A. myc B. fos
C. ras D. Rb

171. Which one of the following is not used as a tumor marker in testicular tumors?

A. AFP B. LDH
C. HCG D. CEA

Ans.	**163. B**	**164. D**	**165. D**	**166. C**	**167. C**	**168. B**
	169. C	**170. A**	**171. D**			

172. A simple bacterial test for mutagenic carcinogens is :

A. Ames test B. Redox test
C. Bacteriophage D. Gene splicing

173. The gene controlling alpah-1-antitrypsin deficiency has been localized to chromosome :

A. 7 B. 14
C. X D. 21

174. A seven-year-old boy has an inherited type of anaemia. He ha an eleven-year-old sister and a fourteen-year-old brother. Both the siblings and both the parents have the trait. The inheritance pattern is :

A. Autosomal dominant B. Autosomal recessive
C. Sex-linked dominant D. Sex-linked recessive

175. All of the following statements about homocystinuria are true except :

A. It is the most common inherited disorder of amino acid metabolism
B. The disorder involves the sulphur-containing amino acids
C. Most patients are mentally retarded
D. Death usually occurs before the first birthday

176. Mother has sickle cell disease; husband is normal : % chances of having, respectively, sickle cell disease and sickle cell trait :

A. 0 and 100 B. 25 and 75
C. 25 and 50 D. 25 and 25

177. All of the following are autosomal dominant disorders except :

A. Tuberous sclerosis B. Polyposis coli
C. Cystic fibrosis D. Myotonia dystonia

178. X-linked recessive disease is characterized by :

A. Vertical transmission
B. 50% female carriers if male is affected
C. 50% male affected if female is diseased
D. 50 % male carriers if female is diseased

179. Which of the following are the eye findings in a case of Trisomy 21 (Down's syndrome)?

1. Palpebral fissure slanting downward medially with prominent epicanthic folds.
2. Brushfield's spots on iris
3. Dislocation of lens
4. Aphakia.

Codes :

A. 1 and 2 B. 2 and 3
C. 3 and 4 D. 1 and 4

Ans.	**172. A**	**173. B**	**174. B**	**175. D**	**176. A**	**177. C**
	178. B	**179. A**				

180. Cri du chat syndrome results due to delection of the short arm of chromosome :

A. 2 B. 3
C. 4 D. 5
E. 6

181. HLA-DR 4 is marker of :

A. Rheumatoid arthritis
B. Sarcoidosis
C. Seronegative gouty arthritis
D. Psoriasis

182. True about autosomal recessive disease except :

A. 25 percent chances in sibling
B. Parents may be normal
C. One of the parents have disease
D. May be severe than many autosomal dominant diseases

183. Carcinoembryonic antigen is seen in :

A. Colorectal carcinoma B. Alcoholic cirrhosis
C. Emphysema D. Diabetes mellitus
E. All of the above

184. True about trisomy 18 syndrome (Edward's) syndrome except :

A. Abnormal vaves
B. Patent ductus arteriosus
C. Ventricular septal defect
D. Normal hands

185. Li fraumeni syndroms is due to :

A. Mutation in the P53 gene
B. Mutation in the ras-oncogene
C. A balanced translocation
D. A multifactorial cause

186. Chromosomal localisation is known in which of the following disorders?

1. Wilson's disease 2. Diabetes mellitus
3. Whipple's disease 4. Retinitis pigmentosa

Select the correct answer using the codes given below :

Codes :

A. 1,2 and 3 B. 1,2 and 4
C. 1,3 and 4 D. 2,3 and 4

187. Gene therapy can be tried in all the following diseases except :

A. Hemophilia A and B B. Turner's Syndrome
C. Phenyl Ketonuria D. HIV—1 disease

Ans.	180. D	181. A	182. C	183. E	184. D	185. A
	186. B	187. B				

188. Which of the following will be the ratio of zygotes produced by a couple both of whom have Bb genotypes at a locus ?

A. 1BB : 1Bb : 1bb B. 2BB : 1Bb : 1 bb

C. 1 BB : 2Bb : 1 bb D. 1BB :2Bb : 2bb

189. Characteristic feature of Klinefeleter's syndrome include :

A. Low levels of gonadotrophin

B. Impotence

C. Gynaecomastia

D. Short stature

E. Congenital heart defects

190. Hellins rule of triplets is :

A. 1 in 40 B. 1 in 80

C. 1 in 802 D. 1 in 803

191. In typical Down's syndrome, the number of ribs is :

A. 9 B. 10

C. 11 D. 12

192. Adrenaline is contraindicated in :

A. Bronchial asthma B. Cardiac asthma

C. Anaphylaxis D. Cardiac arrest

193. In respect of Turner's syndrome, all of the following are true except :

A. Atrial septal defect is the common cardiac abnormality

B. Congenital renal abnormalities are often associated

C. Birth weight is significantly below that of a normal infant

D. Osteoporosis is very often seen

194. All of the following are sex linked diseases except :

A. Hemophilia A B. Hemophilia B

C. Hemophilia C D. Hunter's syndrome

195. HLA antigents are recognised by —— cells :

A. T. Helper B. T-Effector

C. T-Suppressor D. B

196. If both parents have autosomal recessive illnesses, the chances in siblings are :

A. 100% B. 75%

C. 50% D. 25%

197. DNA analysis is done in all except :

A. Hemiphilia A B. Retinoblastoma

C. Sickle cell anemia D. Marfan's syndrome

198. If husband is sexlinked recessive and wife is normal. Which of the following will suffer from the disease :

A. Daughters B. Grand daughters

C. Daughter's sons D. Son's daughters

Ans.	188. C	189. C	190. C	191. C	192. B	193. D
	194. C	195. A	196. A	197. D	198. C	

199. Which of the following does not follow simple Mendelian inhertance :

A. Acute intermittent porphyria
B. Turner's syndrome
C. Tuberous sclerosis
D. Adult polycystic kidney

200. Patau's syndrome is due to :

A. Trisomy 21 B. Trisomy 18
C. 18 p D. Trisomy 13

201. Vitamin D Resistant rickets is interited as :

A. Autosomal dominant B. Autosomal recessive
C. X-linked recessiv D. X-lined dominant

202. Which is an autosomal recessive disease :

A. Marfan's syndrome B. Fabry's disease
C. Noonan's syndrome D. Friedreich's ataxia

203. Which of the following is inherited by single autosomal dominant gene with complete penetrance :

A. Huntigton's chorea B. Albinism
C. Colour blindness D. Schizophrenia

204. HLA associated with hemochromatosis :

A. B27 B. A 3
C. DW 5 D. B 15

205. Laurence Moon Biedl syndrome consists of the following except :

A. Mental retardation B. Retinitis pigmentosa
C. Hypogonadism D. Wasting

206. Polygenic inheritance is seen in :

A. Diabetes mellitus
B. Nephrogenic diabetes insipidus
C. Wilson's disease
D. Rotor's syndrome

207. Feature of Down's syndrome are all except :

A. ↑ Tone
B. Brushfield spots in iris
C. Mild to moderate mental retardation
D. Loose skin at the back of neck

W208. Marfan's syndrome is characterized by the following except :

A. Tall stature B. Arachnodactyly
C. High arched palate D. High arched foot

Ans.	199. B	200. D	201. D	202. D	203. A	204. B
	205. D	206. A	207. A	208. C		

209. Single gene disorder is :

A. Glycogen storage disease
B. Retinoblastoma
C. DM
D. HT

210. A 17-years old girl was seen in the endocrinal clinic with short stature and complaints of amenorrhoea. Examination revealed non development of breast tissue. She was found to have infantile external genitalia. The posterior hairline was low and there were prominent ears with small mandible. She had epicanthal folds, shield chest and cubitus valgus. Most likely chromosomal defect is :

A. XX/XO B. XY/XO
C. XXX D. XYY

211. Which one of the following is not pharmocogenetic :

A. ADA deficiency
B. Warfarin insensitivity
C. Malignant hyperthermia
D. G6PD deficiency

212. A 21-21 translocation was detected in a 25 year old female. What is the chances of her having a normal infant :

A. 100 B. 25
C. 75 D. 0

213. Husband, Wife with 2 children, wife's father had Huntingtons chorea which is true :

A. Chance of getting disease in child is 1 : 4
B. If mother is not affected upto 50 years, there is no chnace of disease in children
C. Wife do not get Huntingtons chorea
D. Huntington chorea is due to point mutation in gere

214. Atavism means similarly with :

A. Grand parents B. His father
C. His mother D. His siblings

215. A defective DNA repair mechanism underlies which of the following conditions except ?

A. Xeroderma pigmentosum
B. Ataxia telangiectasia
C. Bloom syndrome
D. Retinoblastoma

Ans. **209. B** **210. A** **211. A** **212. B** **213. B** **214. A** **215. D**

216. For PCR——— should be known :

A. Gene locus B. Gene morphology

C. Gene sequence D. Gene mutation

217. CA - 125 is found in following except :

A. Mesenchymal Ovarian Ca

B. Endometriosis

C. TB endometritis

D. Stein Levinthal syndrome

218. True in Kawasaki's disease are all except :

A. Fever

B. Occurs above 5 yrs age groups

C. Coronary artery aneurysm

D. Generally benign and self limited

219. 100% recurrence of disease in Down's syndrome :

A. Translocation of 15 + 21 chromsome

B. Mosaic pattern

C. Trisomy - (21, 21 translocation)

D. Non Dysjunction

220. Autosomal recessive with single gene disorder seen in :

A. Wilson disease B. Tuberous sclerosis

C. Neurofibromatosis D. Huntington's chorea

221. Single mutant gene disorder :

A. DM B. RA

C. Glycogen storage ds D. HT

222. In FAP the chromosomal anomaly is seen on :

A. Chr 5 B. Chr 21

C. Chr 6 D. Chr 11

223. HLA matching is not necessary in which of the following organ transplant :

A. Liver B. Bone marrow

C. Pancreas D. Kidney

224. C-erbs B32 gene is responsible for production of :

A. Epidermal growth factor

B. Fibroblast growth factor

C. Tyrosine kinase

D. Transcriptional activators

225. The approximate number of genes contained in the human genome is :

A. 40,000 B. 30,000

C. 80,000 D. 1,00,000

Ans.					
216. C	217. D	218. B	219. C	220. A	221. C
222. A	223. A	224. A	225. D		

226. A married middle aged female gives history of repeated abortions for the past 5 years. The karyotype as given in the examination paper was that of :

A. Klinefeller's syndrome B. Turner's syndrome
C. Down's syndrome D. Patau's syndrome

22'. MHC class III genes encode :

A. Complement component C3
B. Tumor necrosis factor
C. Interleukin - 2
D. Beta 2 microglobulin

228. The HLA class III regions are important elements in :

A. Transplant rejection phenomenon
B. Governing susceptibility to autoimmune diseases
C. Immune surveillance
D. Antigen presentation and elimination

229. Father to son inheritance is never seen in case of :

A. Autosomal dominant inheritance
B. Autosomal recessive inheritance
C. X- linked recessive inheritance
D. Multifactorial inheritance

230. A 48 year old woman was admitted with a history of weakness for two months. On examination, cervical lymph nodes were found enlarged and spleen was palpable 2 cm below the costal margin. Her hemoglobin was 10.5 g/dl, platelet count 237x 109/L and total leukocyte count 40 x 109/L, which included 80% mature lymphoid cells with coarse clumped chromatin. Bone marrow revealed a nodular lymphoid infiltrate. The peripheral blood lymphoid cells were positive for CD19, CD5, CD20 and CD23 and were negtive for CD79B and FMC-7.

Which one of the following statements is not true about this disease?

A. Trisomy 12 correlates an aggressive clinical course
B. Abnormalities of 13q 14 are associated with long term survival
C. Cases with 11q 22-23 deletions have excessive lymph-adenopathy
D. t(11;14) translocation is present in most of the cases.

231. Which of the following inborn errors of metabolism is associated with mental retardation?

A. Alkaptonuria B. Homocystinuria
C. Pentosuria D. Galactosemia

232. Characteristic clinical picture of Maple syrup urine disease :

A. Choreoathetosis B. Flaccid paralysis
C. Petitmal disorder D. Decerebrate rigidity

Ans. 226. C 227. B 228. C 229. C 230. D 231. D 232. D

233. Normal height with decreased bone age is seen in :
A. Cushings syndrome B. Hypothyroidism
C. Thanatotrophic dwarfs D. Down's syndrome

234. Bone age is normal in :
A. Genetic short stature B. Hypopituitarism
C. Hypothyroidism D. Emotional deprivation

235. Herediatry disorders associated with cirrhosis include all except :
A. Amyloidosis B. Galactosemia
C. Cystic fibrosis D. Wilson's disease

236. The following karyotypes are appropriate except :
A. 45, XO 46, XX—Turner mosaic
B. 47, XX—13—Patau's syndrome
C. 46, XY—Noonan's syndrome
D. 47, XYY—Klinefelter's syndrome
E. 45, XX, t (14q21q)—normal female phenotype

237. The following is most diagnostic of Wilson's disease :
A. Kayser-Fleischer ring
B. Low level serum copper
C. Low serum ceruloplasmin
D. Raised SGPT

238. Wilson's disease is characterised by the accumula-tion of copper in :
A. Brain B. Kidney
C. Lung D. All of the above

239. William's syndrome includes all the following except :
A. Small mandible B. Sharp upturned nose
C. Prominent maxilla D. Upward slanting of eyes

240. Commonest malingnancy in a child is :
A. Retinoblastoma B. Renal cell carcinoma
C. Neuroblastoma D. Leukemias

241. Commonest congenital disease in a child is :
A. Down's syndrome B. Klinefelter's syndrome
C. Turner's syndrome D. Cri du chat disease

242. Marfan's syndrome includes :
A. Anophthalmia B. Luxation of lens
C. Spastic muscles D. Congenital dwarfism

243. Which one of the following is usually associated with trisomy 18 syndrome?
A. Polydactyly B. Prominent occiput
C. Micrognathia D. Cleft palate and hare lip
E. Low set ears

Ans.	233. B	234. A	235. A	236. D	237. A	238. D
	239. D	240. D	241. A	242. B	243. D	

244. Which of the following does not belong to trisomy :

A. Down's syndrome B. Patau's syndrome
C. Edward's syndrome D. Pendred's syndrome

245. Infantile body proportions are seen in each of the following conditions except :

A. Cretinism B. Achondroplasia
C. Bowed legs D. Malnutrition

246. Following are features of Turner's syndrome except :

A. Tall stature
B. Cubitus valgus
C. Gonadal dysgenesis
D. Broad chest with wide spaced nipples

247. In Laurence Moon Biedl syndrome, not true is :

A. Pigmentary degeneration
B. Obesity
C. Mental retardation
D. Retinal detachment

248. Osteogenesis imperfecta is :

A. Autosomal dominant B. Autosomal recessive
C. Both A & B D. None of the above

249. Earliest manifestation of Alport's disease is :

A. Microscopic haematuria
B. Proteinuria
C. Oliguria
D. Sensori neural deafness

250. A neonate normal till 5 days of age suddenly threw a seizure and developed irritability with refusal to feed, recurrent hypoglycemia, ketonuria, metabolic acidosis. It could be suffering from :

A. Organic aciduria B. Metabolic acidosis
C. Phenylketonuria D. Alkaptonuria

251. The child of a mother having phenylketonuria with uncontrolled phenylalanine in blood can develop :

A. Phenylketonuria
B. Blond hair with MR
C. MR with cataract
D. Microcephaly, mental retardation and cardiac defects

252. About Down syndrome, following are true except :

A. Decreased Nuchal fold thickness
B. Decreased femur length
C. Decreased humerus length
D. Duodenal atresia

Ans.	244. D	245. B	246. A	247. A	248. C	249. A
	250. A	251. B	252. A			

253. An infant of phenylketonuria presents at 3 weeks, all are true except :

A. Start diet therapy immediately with complete restriction of phenylalanine

B. There will be increased blood phenylalanine and urine phenylacetate levels

C. Tyrosine is an essential amino acid

D. It is diagnosed after institution of protein diet

254. Commonest cause of intestinal obstruction in Down's syndrome is :

A. Duodenal atresia B. Colonic atresia

C. Intestinal atresia D. Oesophageal atresia

255. In the laboratory, for amplification of a single DNA chain, polymerase chain reaction was allowed to continue for 3 cycles. At the end of this, the number of DNA chains would be :

A. 4 B. 8

C. 16 D. 3

256. A neonate was born with cleft lip, cleft palate and cardiac anomalies. There is a history of drugs, which the mother was on. The drug most likely to be implicated :

A. Isotretinoin B. Lithium

C. Valproate D. Phenytoin

257. In triple screening test for Down's syndrome during pregnncy all of the following are included except :

A. Serum beta hCG

B. Serum oestriol

C. Maternal serum Alfa fetoprotein

D. Acetyl cholinesterase

258. The following statements regarding Turner syndrome are true except :

A. Occurrence of Turner syndrome is influenced by material age.

B. Most patients have primary amenorrhoea

C. Most patients have short stature.

D. Edema of hands and feet is an important feature during infancy.

259. A baby girl presents with bilateral inguinal masses, thought to he hernias but are found to be testes in the inguinal canals. Which karyotype would you expect to find in the child?

A. 46, XX B. 46, XY

C. 47, XX D. 47, XYY

Ans. 253. A 254. A 255. B 256. A 257. D 258. A 259. B

260. Dominant gene is :
A. Autosomal B. Sexlinked
C. 100% expressivity D. Always transmitted to offsprings

261. Gene for Huntington's chorea is on :
A. Chromosome 6 B. Chromosome 4
C. Chromosome 19 D. Chromosome 22

262. Philadelphia chromosome refers to :
A. Chromosome 22 B. Chromosome 9
C. Chromosome 12 D. Chromosome 6

263. Philadelphia chromosome is seen in :
A. Chronic myeloid leukaemia
B. Chronic lymphatic leukaemia
C. Acute monocytic leukaemia

264. Least common in Beta thalassemia
A. Gene deletion B. Point mutation
C. Transcription D. Deformity of RNA formation

265. All of the following are chromosomal anomalies except :
A. Down's syndrome B. Edward's syndrome
C. Turner's syndrome D. Haemophilia

266. Edwards syndrome is :
A. Trisomy 21 B. Trisomy 18
C. Trisomy 13 D. 5 p
E. 18 Q

267. Trisomy 21 is seen in :
A. Klinefelter's syndrome B. Down's syndrome
C. Turner's syndrome D. Marfan's syndrome

268. Down's syndrome is due to :
A. Trisomy 21 B. Translocation 13-15/21
C. Translocation 22/21 D. Translocation 22/21
E. All of the above

269. Chances of Down's syndrome are maximum after the age (years) of :
A. 20 B. 30
C. 35 D. 40

270. All are true about Klinefelter's syndrome except :
A. XXY B. Mental retardation seen
C. Infertility D. Short stature

271. A female with chromosomal defect, cubitus valgus, and short neck, is most likely to have :
A. Turner's syndrome B. Klinefelter's syndrome
C. Marfan's syndrome D. Sturge Weber's syndrome

Ans.						
	260. D	261. B	262. A	263. A	264. A	265. D
	266. B	267. B	268. D	269. D	270. D	271. A

272. Chromosomal pattern seen in Turner's syndrome :

A. 45 XO B. 47 XXX

C. Trisomy 21 D. 46 XO

E. Any of the above

273. True about chromosomal abnormalities is :

A. Most of metabolic disorders are chromosomal related

B. Teratoma is genetically governed

C. Alkaptonuria is autosomal dominant

D. Sickle cell anemia is genetically determined with variable penetrance

E. Consanguinity precipitates autosomal recessive disorders

274. Which of the following does not follow simple Mendelian iheritance ?

A. Acute intermittent pophyria

B. Turner's syndrome

C. Tuberous scleosis

D. Adult polycystic kidney

275. All the following features are characteristic of autosomal dominant inheritance of a disease except :

A. Approximately half of the offspring of an affected parent are disesed.

B. Diseased offspring are generally born of consanguinous marriage

C. Both sexes are equally affected

D. If parents are not affected; person may be healthy

276. In autosomal dominant inheritance trait in one of the parent, which will be the inheritance in children :

A. 25% daughters and 75% sons

B. 25% sons and 75% daughters

C. 50% sons and 50% daughters

D. Only in sons

277. Hereditary spherocytosis is :

A. Autosoma dominant B. Autosomal recessive

C. Sex-linked recessive D. Sex-linked dominant

278. An autosoma dominant disease is :

A. Myotonia dystrophica B. Wilson's disease

C. Down's syndrome D. Haemophilia

279. The following genetically determined conditions show an autosoma dominant type of inheritance, except :

A. Tuberous sclerosis B. Cystic fibrosis

C. Polyposis coli D. Dystrophia myotonica

280. Achondroplasia is inherited as :

A. Autosomal recessive B. Autosomal dominant

C. X-linked recessive D. X-linked dominant

Ans.					
272. A	273. E	274. B	275. B	276. C	277. A
278. A	279. B	280. B			

281. **Landouzy-Dejerine muscular dystrophy is transmitted by :**
A. AD B. AR
C. XD D. XR

282. **Autosomal dominant inheritance is seen in all except :**
A. Hepatolenticular degeneration
B. Telangiectasis
C. Huntington's Chorea
D. Achondroplasia

283. **If both parents have autosomal recessive illnesses, the chances in siblings are :**
A. 100% B. 75%
C. 50% D. 25%

284. **True about autosomal recessive disease except :**
A. 25 per cent chances in siblings
B. Parents may be normal
C. Onc of the parents have disease
D. May be severe than many autosomal dominant diseases

285. **Correct about autosomal recessive diseases is that :**
A. One of the parents is involved
B. 50 per cent of siblings are involved
C. Are precipitated by consanguinous marriages
D. They follow Mendelian laws of inheritance

286. **Consangulnous marriages precipitate diseases :**
A. Autosomal dominant B. Autosomal recessive
C. Sex-linked recessive D. Sex-linked dominat

287. **The parents and sons are found to be affected in predigree analysis but there were no consanginous marriages. The chromosomal inheritance is :**
A. Autosomal dominant B. Autosomal recessive
C. X-linked D. Mosacism

288. **Autosomal recessive disease includes:**
A. Cystic fibrosis B. Burton's hypoglobulinemia
C. Black-fair syndrome D. All of the above

289. **An autosomal recessive disease is :**
A. Acute intermittent pophyria
B. Blue-green blindness
C. Hurler's disease
D. Hunter's disease

Ans.	**281. A**	**282. A**	**283. D**	**284. C**	**285. C**	**286. B**
	287. A	**288. D**	**289. A**			

290. All are inherited as autosomal recessive mode of inheritance, except for :

A. Tuberous sclerosis
B. Phenylketonuria
C. Cystic ribosis
D. Friedreich's ataxia
E. Homocystinuria

291. The following disease are transmitted by autosomal recessive genes :

A. Idiopathic haemochromatosis
B. Von Reckling Hausen's disease
C. Von Willebrand disease
D. Cystic fibrosis

292. If husband is sexlinked recessive and wife is normal, which of the following will suffer from the disease :

A. Daughters
B. Grand daughters
C. Daughter's sons
D. Son's daughters

293. X-linked recessive disease is characteised by :

A. Vertical transmission
B. 50% female carriers if male is affected
C. 50% male affected if female is diseased
D. 50% male carriers if female is diseased

294. All sex-linked recessive diseases are :

A. Haemophilia, albinism, red green blindness
B. Haemophilia, albinism, blindness
C. Haemophilia, albinism, blindness G-6-P-D deficiency
D. Haemophilia, blindness, albinism

295. Which of the following is nto a sex-linked disease ?

A. Galactosemia
B. G-6-P-D deficiency
C. Haemophilia
D. Duchenne type of myopathy

296. Which of the following is not an x-linked recessive disease ?

A. Achondroplasia
B. Christmas disease
C. Haemophilia
D. Nephrogenic diabetes insipidus
E. G-6-P-D dehydrogenase deficiency

297. The enzyme G-6-P-D deficiency is :

A. Autosomal dominant
B. Autosomal recessive
C. X-linked dominant
D. X-linked recessive

298. The following are sex-linked inherited diseases :

A. G-6-P-D deficiency
B. Hypogammaglobulinemia
C. Down's syndrome
D. Diamond Blackfan disease
E. Haemophilia

Ans. **290. A** **291. D** **292. D** **293. D** **294. C** **295. A**
296. A **297. D** **298. A,E**

299. Fathers and sons are affected in disease :
A. Autosomal recessive
B. Autosomal dominant with incomplete penetrance
C. X-linked
D. Y-linked

300. Which of the following is not a psychosomatic illness :
A. Bronchial asthma B. Peptic ulcer
C. Venereal disease D. Rheumatoid arthritis

301. Inheritable disease is :
A. Leukaemia B. Aplastic anaemia
C. Myeloma D. Colour blindness

302. Treatable hereditary disorders are :
A. Familial polyposis coli B. Sickle cell disease
C. I.T.P. D. G-6-P-D deficiency

303. Chromosomal anomalies are seen in :
A. Turner's syndrome B. CML
C. All of the above D. Hodgkin's lymphoma

304. Definite chromosomal abnormalites seen in :
A. CML B. Klinefelter's syndrome
C. Bicuspid aortic valve D. All of the above

305. Turner's syndrome include features except :
A. Web neck B. Mental retardation
C. Coarctation of aorta D. Short stature
E. Sexual infantilism

306. Autosomal recessive diseases are except :
A. Wilson's disease B. Phenylketonuria
C. Gaucher's disease D. Galactosemia
E. Gilbert's syndrome

307. Autosomal recessive diseases include :
A. Cystic fibrosis B. Huntington's chorea
C. Marfan's syndrome D. Wilson's disease
E. Hereditary spherocytosis

308. Which of the following is sex-linked?
A. Colour blindness
B. Wilson's disease
C. Duchenne's muscular dystrophy
D. Gilbert's syndrome
E. Marfan's syndrome

309. Following are X-linked except :
A. Haemophilia B. G-6-P-D deficiency
C. Colour blindness D. Fabry's disease
E. Ataxia telangiectasia

Ans.	299. D	300. C	301. D	302. A	303. A,B	304. A,B
	305. B	306. B	307. A,D	308. A,C	309. E	

310. The chromatid division occurs in :

A. Prophase B. Metaphase
C. Interphase D. Telophas

311. In Klinefelter's syndrome, the chromosomal pattern is :

A. XXY B. XXY
C. XO D. Any of the above

312. Disorders with polygenic (Mulitfactorial) inheritance include all, except :

A. Nephrogenic diabetes insipidus
B. Schizophrenia
C. Congenital heart disease
D. Hypertension (essential)

313. With regards to sex hormones, a child with an :

A. XY pattern develops into a normal female
B. XO pattern shows incomplete sexual maturatin puberty
C. XXY pattern develops excessive secondary sexual characters
D. XXY develops into a true hermophrodite

314. The most practical method of preventing genetic disease :

A. Genetic counselling
B. Health Education of masses
C. Premarital checkup
D. Genetic engineering

315. Fanconi's syndrome (Constitutional Aplastic anaemia) is :

A. Autosomal dominant B. Autosomal recessive
C. Sex-linked D. None of the above

316. Klinefelter's syndrome is characterised by :

A. Gynaecomastia
B. Barr-body in buccal smear cells
C. Chromosomal pattern of 47 XXY
D. All of the above

317. HLA are genetically determined and situated on :

A. Chromosome 6 B. Chromosome13
C. Chromosome 18 D. Chromosome 21

318. All diseases are sex-linked except :

A. Haemophilia A B. Haemophilia B
C. Haemophilia C D. Hunter's syndrome

319. X-linked disorders are all except :

A. Haemophilia
B. Familial hypophosphatemic vitamin D refractory rickets
C. Becker type of muscular dystrophy
D. Tuberous sclerosis

Ans.	**310. C**	**311. A**	**312. A**	**313. B**	**314. A**	**315. B**
	316. D	**317. A**	**318. C**	**319. D**		

320. Impotency is not uncommon in all except :

A. Klinefelter's syndrome
B. Familial trait
C. Diabetes mellitus
D. Acromegaly

321. The characteristic feature of klinefelter's syndrome includes :

A. Short stature
B. Gynaecomastia
C. Low gonadotrophin level
D. Congenital heart defect

322. All of the following are associated with abnormality of chromosomal number, except :

A. Klinefelter's syndrome
B. "Le cri du chat" (cat cry) syndrome
C. Turner's syndrome
D. XXY constitution

323. Y-linked dominant condition is :

A. Vitamin D resistant rickets
B. Hemophilia
C. Hairy ears
D. Nephrogenic diabetes insipidus

324. Huntington's chorea is :

A. Autosomal dominant B. Autosomal recessive
C. X-linked recessive D. Y-linked dominant

325. Warfan's syndroem involves all of the following except :

A. Abnormalities of eyes B. Long tapering fingers
C. Marked obesity D Dissecting aneurysm

326. One of the following is the characteristic feature of Down's syndrome :

A. Macroglossia B. Mental retardation
C. Single palmar crease D. All of the above

327. All of the following are autosomal dominant, except :

A. Achondroplasia B. Neurofibromatosis
C. Von Willebrand's disease
D. Wilson's disease

328. Which of the following is not transmitted by simple Mendellan inheritance ?

A. Marfan's syndrome
B. Truner's syndrome
C. Acute intermittent porphyria
D. Adult polycystic kidney

Ans.						
	320. A	321. B	322. B	323. C	324. A	325. C
	326. A	327. D	328. B			

329. The Philadelphia chromosome is an acquired chromosomal abnormality associated with :

A. Acute meloid leukaemia
B. Chronic myeloid leukaemia
C. Acute lymphatic leukaemia
D. Chronic lymphatic leukaemia

330. X-linked recessive disorders include all, except :

A. Christmas disease
B. Duchenne muscular dystrophy
C. Nephrogenic diabetes insipidus
D. Osteogenesis imperfecta

331. Regarding vitamin D resistant rickets all are true, except :

A. Is an X-linked dominant disorder
B. Is resistant to oridinary therapeutic doses of vitamin D
C. The disease persists even adult life and causes osteomalacia
D. Treatment consists of small doses of vitamin D

332. Match the following ;

I. Vitamin D resistant rickets	(i) Autosomal recessive
II. Haemophilia	(ii) Autosomal dominant
III. Albinism	(iii) X-linked dominant
IV. Huntington's chorea	(iv) X-linked recessive

A. I (i)	II (ii)	III (iii	IV (iv)
B. I (ii)	II (i)	III (iv)	IV (iii)
C. I (iv)	II (iii)	III (i)	IV (ii)
D. I (iv)	II (iii)	III (ii)	IV (i)

333. In Marfan's syndrome all are seen, except :

A. Long thin extremeties
B. Dissecting aneurysm
C. Marked obesity
D. Changes in the eyes

334. Galactosaemia is characterised by :

A. Cataract formation
B. Mental retardation
C. Cirrhosis
D. All of the above

335. Increased risk of all the following genetic disorders are seen in mothers over 40 years old, except :

A. Down's syndrome
B. Turner's syndrome
C. Klinefelter's syndrome
D. Edward's syndrome

336. Turner's syndrome is :

A. Autosomal dominant
B. Autosomal recessive
C. Chromosomal abberant
D. Y-linked disease

Ans.					
329. B	330. D	331. D	332. C	333. C	334. D
335. B	336. C				

337. **Short stature is not seen in :**
A. Achondroplasia B. Dwarfism
C. Marfan's syndrome D. Turner's syndrome

338. **A Notable example of X-linked dominant disorder is :**
A. Duchenne muscular dystrophy
B. Glucose-6-Phosphate dehydrogenase deficiency
C. Vitamin D resistant rickets
D. Nephrogenic diabetes insipidus

339. **Wilson's disease, an autosomal recessive disorder is characterized by all, except :**
A. Excessive deposits of copper in liver cells (cirrhosis)
B. Degenerative changes in the brain (hepatolenticular disease)
C. Pathognomonic greenish brown ring (kayser-Fieischer ring) at the limus of cornea
D. Increased hepatic synthesis of copper binding alpha 2-globulin (ceruloplasmin)

340. Spider fingers A. Turner's syndrome
341. Coarctation of aorta B. Osteogenesis imperfecta
342. Epicanthic folds C. Ehler Danlos syndrome
343. Blue sclera D. Marfan's syndrome
344. Hyper extensibility of skin E. Mongolism

ChromosomeChromosome abnormality-Clinical syndrome

345. Trisomy - 13 A. Down's
346. Trisomy - 18 B. Wolf's
347. Trisomy - 21 C. Patau's
348. 4 p D. Edwards
349. 5p E. Cri du chat

350. Autosomal dominant A. Vitamin D resistant rickets
351. Autosomal recessive B. No proven examples
352. X-linked recessive C. Duchenne muscular dystrophy
353. X-linked dominant D. Limb girdle muscular dystrophy (Erb)
354. Y-lined inheritance E. Myotonic dystrophy

355. **These statements regarding human chromosomes are correct, except :**
A. There are 46 chromosomes
B. Each gamete contains 46 chromosomes
C. The haploid number is 23
D. There are 2 sex chromosomes
E. Most common type of aneuploidy is trisomy

Ans. 337. C 338. C 339. D 340. D 341. A 342. E 343. B 344. C
345. C 346. D 347. A 348. B 349. E 350. E 351. D 352. C
353. A 354. B 355. B

356. Genotype is :
A. Physical characteristics
B. Physical & genetic characteristics
C. Physiological 7 genetic characteristics
D. Total genetic constitution

357. Philadelphia chromosome is present in 90% cases of :
A. CML B. AML
C. CLL D. Acute monocytic leukaemia

358. Down's syndrome is due to :
A. Chromosomal abnormality B.Endocrine abnormality
C. Metabolic disorder D. None of the above

359. Down's syndrome is trisomy of chromosome :
A. 5 B. 12
C. 21 D. 22

360. Mongolism is closely associated with :
A. Duration of gestation B. Rubella during pregnancy
C. Spacing D. Maternal age

361. Down's syndrome occurs in females of :
A. Early marriages B. Late marriages
C. Polycystic ovaries D. Short statured

362. The changes of Down's syndrome are maximum if age of the mother is :
A. 18 years B. 21 years
C. 30 years D. 40 years

363. A child with 21-trisomy has these characteristics, except :
A. Hypertonia
B. Mental regardation
C. Oblique palpebral fissures
D. Simian crease
E. Incurving little fingers

364. Correct about Down's syndrome is :
A. Commonest cause of mental retardation
B. ↓ Epicanthic folds
C. Incidence is 1 in 1500
D. Rudimentary acetabulum

365. All the following are features of Down's syndrome except :
A. Respiratory tract infections
B. Clinodactyly
C. Hypotonia
D. Pigmented birth marks

Ans.	**356. D**	**357. A**	**358. A**	**359. C**	**360. D**	**361. B**
	362. D	**363. A**	**364. A**	**365. D**		

366. Infants with Down's syndrome can have :

A. Pyloric stenosis B. Annular pancreas
C. Hirschsprung's disease D. Duodenal atresia

367. Which of the following has increased incidence in Down's syndrome ?

I. Endocardial cushion defect
II. Duodenal atresia
III. Anorectal anomaly
IV. Renal disease

A. I, II, III, IV B. I, III, IV
C. II, III, IV D. II, IV

368. Hypertelorism is found in :

A. Down's syndrome B. Gargolysim
C. Turner's syndrome D. None of the above

369. In Down's syndrome, there is increased risk of :

A. Leukaemia B. Heart defects
C. Megacolon D. Meckel's diverticulum

370. Which one of the following is usually not associated with trisomy 18 syndrome ?

A. Polydactly B. Prominent occiput
C. Micrognathia D. Cleft palate and hare lip
E. Low set ears

371. An infant with 18-trisomy has the following features, except :

A. Normal intelligence B. Flexion of the fingers
C. Rocker-bottom feet D. Prominent occiput
E. Micrognathia

372. Klinefelter's syndrome is a :

A. Metabolic disorder B. Psychological disorder
C. Chromosomal disorder D. Malignant disorder

373. Chromosomal pattern in Klinefelter's syndrome :

A. 45 XO B. 46 XY
C. 47 XXY D. 47 XYY

374. All are true in Klinefelter's syndrome except :

A. XXY pattern B. Gynaecomastia
C. Mental retardation D. Short stature

375. In Turner's syndrome which of the following are seen ?

A. Short stature
B. Streaky gonads
C. Chromosomal constitution XO
D. Chromosomal (Mosaic) XX
E. All of the above

Ans.	366. C,D	367. A	368. A	369. A,B	370. D	371. A
	372. C	373. C	374. D	375. E		

376. Which match is not true ?

A. Wilson's disease : Ceruloplasmin
B. Chromosome 5 : Cri du chat syndrome
C. Phenylketonuria : Phenylalanine hydroxylase
D. Turner's syndrome : XXY

377. Turner's syndrome is characterized by all except :

A. Short stature
B. Gonadal agenesis
C. Prominent nipples
D. Cubitus valgus

378. Turner's syndrome is usually associated with all of the following clinical features, except :

A. Short stature
B. Gonadal dysgenesis
C. Mental retardation
D. Primary amenorrhoea
E. Broad chest with wide spaced nipple

379. A child with microcephaly, epicanthic folds and mewing cry is suggestive of :

A. Cretinism
B. Edward's syndrome
C. Down's syndrome
D. Cri du chat syndrome

380. Which is not a feature of Pierre-Robbin syndrome ?

A. Respiratory distress
B. Mandibular hypoplasia
C. Coloboma irides
D. Hearing defect

381. In autosomal dominant inheritance trait in one of the parent, which will be inheritance in children ?

A. 25% daughters and 75% sons
B. 25% sons and 75% daughters
C. 50% daughters and 50% sons
D. Only in sons

382. Hereditary spherocytosis is :

A. Autosomal dominant
B. Autosomol recessive
C. Sex-linked recessive
D. Sex-linked dominant

383. Characteristic of autosomal recessive inheritance :

A. 25%
B. 50%
C. 15%
D. 75%
E. None of the above

384. Cystic fibrosis is :

A. Autosomal dominant
B. Autosomal recessive
C. X-linked recessive
D. X-linked

Ans.	**376. D**	**377. C**	**378. C**	**379. D**	**380. C**	**381. C**
	382. A	**383. A**	**384. B**			

385. True about sex linked recessive disease in a male whose wife is not a carriers is that the following will have the disease :

A. Son's daugthers B. Daughter's sons
C. Daughters D. Sons

386. True regarding X linked recessive transmission is :

A. Vertical transmission
B. Affected male transmits to 50% of his sons
C. 50% of daughters of carrier females are affected
D. 50% of male children of female carrier affected..

387. All of the following are X-linked recessive conditions, except :

A. Nephrogenic Diabetes insipidus
B. Haemophilia
C. G-6-P-d deficiency
D. Myotonia congentia

388. The only Y-linked disease is :

A. Cystic fibrosis B. Haemophilia
C. Colour blindness D. Hairy ears

389. Infantile body proportions are seen in each of the following conditions except :

A. Cretenism B. Achondroplasia
C. Bowed legs D. Malnutrition

390. Each of the following conditions can be diagnosed by amniocentesis except :

A. Fetal sex B. Down's syndrome
C. Cretinism D. R. incompatibility

391. Marfan's syndrome is characterized by the following except :

A. Mental retardation B. Subluxation of lens
C. Arachnodactyly D. C.V.S. disorder

392. A child with blue sclera and multiple fractures has :

A. Rickets B. Scurvy
C. Osteogenesis imperfecta D. Achondroplasia

393. A child with old healed fractures with blue sclera and now complains of bone pains has :

A. Leukaemia B. Scurvy
C. Osteogenesis imperfecta D. Osteodystrophy

394. Osteogenesis impertecta is associated with :

A. Blue sclera B. Red hair
C. White nail D. White line

395. Aminocentesis done in following conditions :

A. Down's syndrome B. Anencephaly
C. Muscular dystrophy D. Haemophilia

Ans.	385. B	386. D	387. D	388. D	389. B	390. C
	391. A	392. C	393. C	394. A	395. ALL	

396. Chromosomal abnormality seen in all except :
A. G-6-P-D deficiency
B. CML
C. Polycystic kidney disease
D. Turner's syndrome
E. von Willebrand's disease

397. An infant with 18-trisomy has the following features except :
A. Normal intelligence
B. Flexion of the fingers
C. Rocker-bottom feet
D. Prominent occiput
E. Micrognathia

398. A child with 21-trisomy has following characteristics :
A. Hypertonia
B. Mental retardation
C. Oblique palpebral fissures
D. Simian crease
E. Incurving little fingers

399. Coarctation of aorta is commonly associated with :
A. Down's syndrome
B. Turner's syndrome
C. Aortic stenosis
D. Congenital rubella

400. Turner's syndrome is characterized by :
A. Gonadal dysgenesis
B. ↑ Gonadotrophins
C. Normal gonadotrophins
D. Short stature
E. Mental retardation

401. Autosomal recessive inheritance :
A. Manifests if dominant
B. Severe in homozygotes
C. 25% of children are carriers if both parents heterozygotes
D. 5% of children are normal if both parents heterozygotes
E. 50% are heterozygotes

402. Autosomal recessive disease are :
A. Galactosaemia
B. Cystic fibrosis
C. Phenylketonuria
D. Christmas disease
E. Achondroplasia

403. X-linked diseases are :
A. Hemophilia
B. G-6-P-D deficiency
C. Christmas disease
D. Colour blindness
E. Duchenne type of myopathy

404. X-linked dominant diseases are :
A. Hyper phosphataemic rickets
B. Incontinentia pigmenti
C. Oro facial digital syndrome
D. Achondroplasia

Ans.					
	396. A	**397. A**	**398. A**	**399. B**	**400. A,B,D**
	401. B,C,D	**402. A,B,C**	**403. ALL**	**404. A,B,C**	

MATCHING

405.	47/XXY	A.	Mongolism
406.	**47/XXX**	B.	Super female
407.	**47/21 Trisomy**	C.	Turner's syndrome
408.	**45/XO**	D.	Klinefelter's syndrome
409.	**Trisomy-18**	E.	Edward's syndrome
410.	**Streak gonads**	A.	Wolf's syndrome
411.	**Low ridge count of digits**	B.	Patau's syndrome
412.	**Polydactyly**	D.	Turner's syndrome
413.	**Rocker bottom feet**	E.	EDward's syndrome
414.	**Coloboma**		

TRUE (T) OR FALSE (F)

415. **Philadelphia chromosome is seen in acute myeloid leukaemia.**
416. **A girl with Turner's syndrome may be 45, XX.**
417. **Sex-chromatin or 'Barr-body' which represents a genetically inactive X chromosome.**
418. **As with autosomal recessive conditions, the heterozygons carrier is usually diseased.**
419. **Duchenne muscular dystrophy is sex-linked inheritance disease transmitted solely by healthy female carriers.**
420. Autosomal recessive genes manifest their clinical effect only in homozygotes.
421. Mental retardation is not common in Down's syndrome.
422. Only males are clinically affected in X linked recessive disorders.
423. Patients with Down's syndrome have Trisomy
424. The frequency or acute lymphoblastic leukaemia is high with Down's syndrome
425. Mental retardation is a prominent feature of Turner's syndrome
426. Klinefelter's syndrome is associated with advanced maternal age.
427. Mental regardation appears to increase with increase number of X chromosomes.
428. Fragile X syndrome may or may not be associated with macro-orchidism in males.
429. Cleft lip and palate is a multifactorial inheritacne abnormality

THOUGHT PROVOKING QUESTIONS

Directions : *Fill in with the most appropriate words and check your power of comprehension. (The answers are provided at the end)*

430. **Melnick-needles syndrome of multiple malformations is inherited as...**
431. Euploid cells with more than teh normal diploid number of 46 chromosomes are termed..

Ans.	405. D	406. B	407. A	408. C	409. E	410. D
	411. C	412. B	413. E	414. A		

432. Majority of translocation leading to Down's syndrome consist of centric fusion of chromosomes between ...
433. The chromosomes affected in this deletion syndrome causing low bith weight, mental retardation and cat like cry is ....
434. Deletion of this chromosome is associated with Wilm's tumor...
435. Dermatoglyphic feature or large size dermal pattern on the digits is characteristic of this chromosmal abberatin....
436. Syndrome consisting of phenotypic features resulting from a sex chromosome complement that includes two or more X chromosomes and one or more Y chromosomes is...
437. The most frequent chromosomal abberation found among the products of spontaneous abortion is ....
438. Prenatal diagnosis by amniocentesis is usually undertaken at gestation of...
439. The most important clinical indications for chromosomal study is ....

THOUGHT PROVOKING QUESTIONS

Directions : *Fill in with the most appropriate words and check your power of comprehension. (The answers are provided at the end of these questions).*

440. Main disadvantage of chorionic villous biopsy which scores over aminocentesis in almost all aspects
441. Chromosomal disorder showing increased icnidence of diabetes mellitus...
442. The most common abnormalities in the number of autosomes in a live born infant is ....
443. Menke's syndrome is a X linked recessive disorder. The defect here is block in ...
444. The enzyme that is lacking in ochronosis....
445. The single most cause of primary amenorrhoea...
446. An autosomal dominant disease characterised by a variety of benign and malignant neoplasms, widely spread throughout the body especially retinal and cerebellar hemangiomas..
447. Retinitis pigmentosa, mental retardation skull deformities, syndactyly and polydactyly...
448. Brush field's spots is a distinctive ocular feature seen in patients with ...
449. Genetic information is more extensive on...
450. Male chromatin body or F-body or extensive on..
451. The most frequent source for study of Barr bodies...
452. Chromosomal analysis (ingrowing cells) is Barr bodies...
453. The most freqeunt is ...
    Chromosomal defects as a whole are...
    I. Autosomal....
    II. Sex chromosomal...

454. With live births, trisomy of sex chromosomes is most frequent chromosomal anamoly as a whole...

455. With live births, the most frequent autosomal anomaly is ...

456. A reliable marker for the impending 'blast phase' in CML is appearance of an isochromosome for the logn arm of ...

457. The prognosis for a ML with a triad of translocation (Auer bodies and decreased leukocyte, Alkaline phosphatase) is....

458. The chromosomal abnormality in normal female with metnal retardation is ....

459. Hurler's syndrome is differentiated from Hunter's syndrome by ...

460. Among the offspring of consanguineous matings there is an increased perinatal mortality rate together with an increased frequency of both...

461. The normal and abnormal genes (alternative forms of the same gene) are known as .....

462. Usually children born to XXX females are ....

463. The use of DNA marker is important in detecting autosomal disorders before symptoms and signs are evident and in antenatal diagnosis. The diagnosis depends on demonstrating that the disease gene is lined to .....

464. The process of random inactivation of the X chromosome is referred as.....

(Answers 415-464)

415. F	**416. F**	**417. T**
418. F	**419. T**	**420. T**
421. F	**422. T**	**423. T**
424. T	**425. F**	**426. T**
427. T	**428. T**	**429. T**

430. X-linked Dominant Inheritance

431. Polypoid

432. No. 21 and 13, 14, 15

433. 5p-

434. Chromosome 21

435. Turner's syndrome

436. Klinefelter syndrome

437. 45 X karyotype

438. 15-16 weeks

439. Multiple congenital malformations with mental retardation of unkown origin, deceased infant

440. It can not screen for neural tube defects

441. Turner's syndrome

442. Trisomy 21 (Down's syndrome)

443. Intestinal absorption of copper

444. Homogenistic acid defect

445. Gonadal dysgenesis
446. Von Hippel Lindaue disease
447. Lawrence Moon Biedl syndrome
448. Down's syndrome
449. X-chromosome
450. Y-chromosome
451. Desquamated cells
452. Late Prophase
453. I. Autosomal Trisomy 18 (commonest) Triploidy
II. Sex chromosomal - 45 XO (Turner's syndrome)
454. Klinefelter's syndrome (XXY)
455. Down's syndrome
456. Chromosome 17 (17q)
457. Good
458. 48 XXXX
459. Clouding o the cornea
460. Congenital annomalies and mental retardation
461. Alleles
462. Normal
463. RFLP's (Restriction Fragment Length Polymorphisms)
464. Lyonisation